Practical Reiki

Practical Reiki

Dr Mari Hall

Thorsons
An Imprint of HarperCollins*Publishers*

Thorsons
An Imprint of HarperCollins*Publishers*
77–85 Fulham Palace Road,
Hammersmith, London W6 8JB
1160 Battery Street
San Francisco, California 94111–1213

Published by Thorsons 1997
10 9 8 7 6 5 4

A catalogue record for this book
is available from the British Library

ISBN 0 7225 3465 5

Printed in Great Britain by Woolnough Bookbinding Ltd.

Dedication

This book is dedicated to the innocence and purity of all souls, the radiant light that is alive in all beings. It is my vision that we remember that we are one family, and go forth together to create a world of peace. It is time to give our future generations a heritage of LOVE.

'Your hands can be the instrument
for the peace and well-being of
your family, friends, yourself
and our world.'

Mari Hall

Contents

Acknowledgements

It is my heartfelt joy to acknowledge:

My many students and clients who have walked beside me and allowed me to be a silent witness to their miracles.

K. Bradford Brown and J. Roy Whitten, co-founders of 'The Life Training', who taught me to listen to my mind, feel with my heart and, most importantly, to live LIFE fully.

Baba, who has given me many experiences, and taught me that hope is what keeps faith from drying out, and that faith and hope together are the midwife of Love.

My family: it is because of their full support and love, that I have been able to reach for the stars!

An Important Foreword

To give first or second degree Reiki, or to be a Reiki practitioner or Master of Reiki, requires that you receive attunements *in person* from a Reiki Master Teacher who has themselves received the attunements and training. This book can never be regarded as a substitute for that direct initiation process.

It was written to be informative, with the express desire to give you an understanding of Reiki and how it can be used, and to open up to you the possibility that you too could be an instrument for this loving energy. Once you have been initiated by a Reiki Master who has been properly trained, this book can be used as a guide for you to do your work.

Introduction

You are about to begin a special journey as you read this book. It is my hope that it will awaken you to the possibility that you can also reach out and help people or yourself, and be touched by one of the highest forms of energy that exists. It originated in Tibet over 3,000 years ago and has been passed down through the centuries. Reiki is not hard to learn; in fact, it is the most simple therapeutic method I know of. It possesses a unique wisdom of its own, directing itself to where it is most needed. No special medical knowledge is necessary in order to practise Reiki. It can be used to complement all other healing methods. It is so simple to use – all you need is your hands to transfer this energy. Often immediate relief is obtained for all kinds of complaints. It has been my experience that the healing and harmonizing effects of Reiki involve not only the recipient, but the instrument (the person giving the Reiki) as well, leaving them both filled with peace, joy and vitality.

When I first became a Reiki Master, I wrote manuals for my students to use in the seminars. It was very important to me that the manuals should contain the purest essence of Reiki and be presented with integrity. I spent months compiling the information and writing the text. Each manual is an integral part of the Reiki courses I teach. As time has gone by, I have changed, and the manuals have changed too. They have undergone three major revisions. The pure essence of Reiki is still there, supplemented by other information I have come across and found useful. The latest material from my course manuals is included in this book. The history of Reiki that is found in Chapter 1 is the one told to me by my Reiki Master; it contains many spiritual principles that have helped me on my life's journey. *Practical Reiki* was written in the hope that more and more people will know about this wonderful natural healing method. It is my desire that somewhere in these pages, you will be encouraged to take a Reiki course in order to use this technique with your family, friends and yourself, or to have a Reiki treatment. I can truly say that, either way, there is usually a feeling of having experienced something beautiful. Your heart will open and, as a result of this experience, something within will be transformed.

Reiki is not in the mind; it is in the heart. Feeling it is always the greatest teacher.

About Myself and My Vision

A trusted friend and teacher, K. Bradford Brown, asked me many years ago how I wanted the world to be. During a meditation I had a vision for the world. My eyes were closed, yet I could see the world as we might see it from space. All around the world were people holding hands. They were brothers and sisters. We had respect for our differences – all the things that made us the wonderful, unique individuals that we are. It did not matter that we had different skin colours, philosophies and languages, because we had something that overcame all these things and united us. It was LOVE and there was peace in our world.

I realized that, in order to have peace outside of me, it had to start within me first. I began my search for that something that would bring me peace, and hopefully, health. I had been reading about and studying religion and different philosophies, thinking that if I came back to a spiritual centre-point my problems would be solved. I had been awarded a doctorate in divinity, yet my health, both physically and emotionally, was still not good. I was divorced from my husband and had taken a powerful course called 'The Life Training', which had originated in California, in the USA. This had been a big turning point in my life. The training gave me the tools to cease living my life from the conditioned reactions of my mind, and to respond to life with love.

Throughout my early life, I was constantly 'down' with something. I had all sorts of illnesses. I spent a good part of my married life in and out of hospitals and having major surgery. I heard about Reiki and was ready! I became so convinced that this was my life path that I became a Reiki Master. Over the years, Reiki has deepened my spiritual experience and in 1988 I was ordained as a minister of religion and counsellor. It has given me health and vitality so that I have never since been hospitalized. I travel and teach Reiki to people of many different countries and cultures who are searching for something with meaning in their lives – a way to be active in their own health and in the health of others.

The vision I had many years ago is still alive in me. It is in my mind and heart. It is the motivation to continue my work for world peace with the use of Reiki. I designed a symbol to represent this vision. It is a symbol I wear all the time and I am sharing it with you:

It is called 'The Heart of the Family' and is also the symbol for the members of The International Association of Reiki. The people on the outside of the drawing represent the people all around the world holding hands – the brothers and sisters. The heart represents the love and respect that we have for each other and for ourselves. The baby represents the innocence and purity of our souls – the Light. We are the heart of the family; each of us is important and integral to each other and to our world.

I welcome you to join with us in this vision of a peaceful, love-filled world, starting with ourselves and spreading out to all humanity.

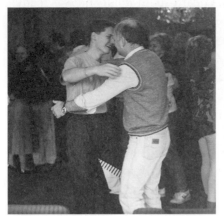

Figure 1

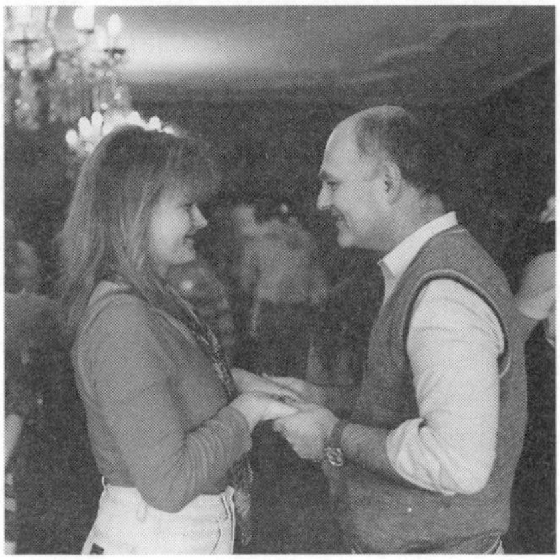

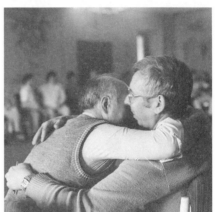

Figure 2

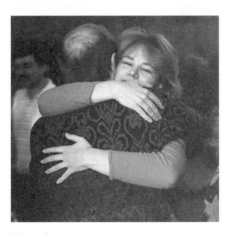

Figure 3

Figure 4

Photographs from a Reiki seminar lead by Mari

What is Reiki?

Reiki is a Japanese word and is pronounced 'Ray-Key'.

Figure 5: Hawayo Takata's calligraphy for Reiki

Running style used by the Reiki Alliance.

There are many styles of calligraphy for writing Japanese characters. These are the normal ways to see Reiki written (Figure 5). The first is an actual copy of Hawayo Takata's calligraphy and the other is the style commonly used by the Reiki Alliance (another international organization of Reiki). Both are Japanese calligraphy for Reiki.

'Rei' is defined as Universal life giving and, like the rays of the sun, it gives life to living things. It is all-knowing; a spiritual consciousness. 'Ki' is defined as energy: this energy or life force flows through all things that are alive. 'Ki' is also known as Light, Prana, Chi, Cosmic Energy, or Universal Radiant Energy.

Reiki is Universal Life-giving Energy and can be used for all purposes, conditions and situations. It can be safely used at any time, in any place and for anything. To practise Reiki, no faith or belief is required. It is successfully used by people of many differing religions, philosophies and ages. It is for everyone. Reiki is the most simple natural healing method I know of. Once a person is reawakened by a Reiki Master with an initiation process, then the ability to transmit this energy will be theirs for the rest of their lives and will flow through their hands naturally.

5

It is my belief that we are all born with this Universal Life Energy, but that our reactions to life cause us to become less open, with the result that the natural flow of energy is less pure and less available. Our personality, that is our ego or false self, is the filter for the energy. Practising Reiki can enable us to shift into a harmonious state that is often referred to as an alpha or theta state of consciousness. In these states of being, the filter aspect is harmonized, returning us to our natural wholeness. We are open to the divine moment of love and healing.

What Reiki Is Not

Reiki is not mind-directed energy, polarity therapy or therapy using magnetism. With these approaches, the therapist must see the energy coming into them and direct it with their minds. In these approaches to healing, illness is considered as negative energy. The therapist, who is filled with positive energy, attracts the negative energy like a magnet, pulling it away and removing it from the client. One of the biggest fears is that the negative energy from the client will somehow attach itself to the therapist, making them ill. Or conversely, there is concern that, if the therapist has negative energy, it could be picked up by the client.

What Reiki Is

With Reiki, you do not have to see the energy, nor concentrate on it at all. Nor do you remove energy from someone, or give them your energy. Reiki energy balances and harmonizes. If there is too much energy in an area, or if there is not enough, the area is out of balance: when there is imbalance, there is potential for illness. In a balanced state, the individual has the potential for self-healing. The energy is transmitted simply by placing your hands on yourself or another individual.

We do not diagnose with Reiki. Rather, we understand that the body is in a state of balance or imbalance. Reiki makes its way to the areas of imbalance during a treatment. No medical or diagnostic education is required. Reiki works on many levels of living things. The physical, mental, emotional and spiritual aspects are all enhanced with Reiki energy.

Energy is all around us and inside us as well. We constantly react and respond to energy without realizing it, all day, every day. Around us is an energy field which is referred to as the aura. The aura has many levels: emotional, mental and spiritual levels. Surrounding the Universe is an aura with layers as well. One of these layers is called Universal, Unconditional Love. Reiki is the Unconditional Love of the Universe. If you are a religious person and believe that God, or that Universal divine essence, by what ever name it is called, created the Universe, it can then be thought that Reiki is the Unconditional Love of God or that divine essence.

Reiki is given from the heart and is often experienced as the receiving of unconditional love. This love has the power to bring us back to a state of peace and harmony. This state can be described as health or wholeness. For many people, giving and receiving this energy is a spiritual experience, because we experience 'wholeness', which is holy. It is impossible for me to separate holiness from Reiki. It has been my continued experience as a Reiki Master, an instrument and recipient of this energy, that wholeness is a feeling and expression of 'being one' with all living things.

Illness is the result of imbalance. The cause of the illness can usually be found at a deeper level of the emotional, mental or spiritual aspects. For instance, if you always lived your life in fear, the imbalance could occur in different areas of your body. One is the solar plexus region, as fear usually constricts energy there (producing, for example, a tight, cold stomach). You could also have constricted energy in the throat area, from not expressing yourself. The potential for illness will always be greater in areas of imbalance.

When I was a young girl, a series of incidents happened which influenced me in making a decision not to trust anyone or anything. This was a mental decision which was based on an emotional reaction. As a result, I had chronic throat problems throughout my life. Imbalance created illness. Because the Reiki energy works on all levels, the cause is being treated as well as the resulting illness.

Most importantly, people who transmit Reiki energy are not healers; they are instruments for this energy. The person who receives the energy is harmonized so that their body can heal itself naturally. They are empowered in their healing process. There is a natural relationship, a partnership. The recipient is always the healer.

Also, as you transmit this energy you are being harmonized at the same time. You are receiving a treatment as you are giving one. The more you use Reiki, the better it becomes, because you are becoming more harmonized. The more balanced you are, the better the energy will be.

Chapter 1
The History of Reiki

The story of Reiki has been passed from master to student for many years. This is how it was told to me by my Reiki Master.

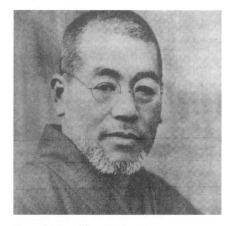

Figure 6: Dr Mikao Usui.

Dr Mikao Usui was the dean of a small Christian university in Kyoto, Japan. One day, during a discussion with some of his students, he was asked if he believed in the literal translation of the Bible and, specifically, if he believed in the miracles of healing performed by Christ. His reply was 'Yes'. The next question startled Dr Usui because they asked him why, if Christ had said 'You will do as I have done, and even greater things', how come there were not more healers in the world.

Then they asked him to teach them the methods that Christ had used to heal. Bound by his honour in traditional Japanese style, he resigned his position as dean because he could not give them their answers. He

9

was determined to find the answers to this great mystery and turned to the USA as the first place to seek answers to these questions. Because he was a Christian missionary and minister, he studied at the University of Chicago. During his seven years of study in America, he tried to understand through Scripture how Jesus effected miracles and transformation. During this time, Dr Usui received a doctorate in theology, but he did not find the revelations he was seeking. He travelled to Northern India and Tibet, since it was said that Christ had studied there. It was during this time that he learned Sanskrit, the ancient and sacred language of the Hindus. He studied the Tibetan Lotus Sutras and felt that he had found the intellectual answers to the mystery of Christ's healing, but not the empowerment. Dr Usui returned to Japan and began to focus on the Buddha. He realized that the Buddha had performed the same miracles as Jesus. He too healed the sick and had a great control of energy, because he channelled the power of God and the Universe. Dr Usui began to question the different Buddhist sects concerning their ability to perform the miracles that Buddha performed: could they heal the body? The Buddhists said they did not believe that the healing of the body and spirit were always directly related. They concentrated their energy on the spirit and left the healing of the body to those concerned with the healing arts. They believed that the body and the spirit were separate, and that it was the spirit that needed healing.

Dr Usui's journey led him finally to a Zen monastery. He asked the head monk the same question: 'Do you know how to heal the body?' The monk replied, 'Not anymore.' This answer puzzled Dr Usui, so he pursued, 'What do you mean, not anymore?' The monk explained that so much emphasis had been placed on healing the spirit that they had forgotten the body, but also emphasized that what was ever possible at one time could be accomplished again. Dr Usui was so elated with the monk's enthusiasm that he asked for his help in his quest to rediscover how to heal the body. He was admitted to the Zen monastery in Tokyo and began to study under the guidance of the Zen monk. During his years at the monastery, he read the Sutras, the writings and teachings of Buddha, but did not find the answer. Many times, he sought the guidance of the Zen monk, who always told Dr Usui to meditate, for in meditating he would find the answer within.

Through meditation, Dr Usui was guided to learn Chinese. It was during this time of study that he began to find what he considered to be the secret of empowerment for healing. He found what he believed to be the keys that would open the way to healing of the kind Christ and Buddha had once performed.

Dr Usui returned to the monk to share his findings and seek guidance. Through meditation, he and the monk were told he should go to a holy mountain near Kyoto, called Kuri Yama. While on the mountain, he was to fast and meditate for twenty-one days. During this time he would receive enlightenment and spiritual clarity.

Dr Usui made the pilgrimage from Tokyo to Kuri Yama, with a few belongings. At the top of the mountain, he found a location facing the East. Each morning, he would rise before the sun and throw away one of the twenty-one stones he had placed in front of his place of meditation. Each day, he meditated and fasted. When Dr Usui awakened on the twenty-first day, he could not even see his hand in front of his face. It was like a new moon day, when no light shines in the heavens before the breaking of dawn. Dr Usui found his way to his meditation place and picked up the last stone. Before throwing the last stone off the side of the mountain, he prayed. He asked God for confirmation of his findings and asked to receive enlightenment to show him how to use them.

As he threw the stone off the side of the mountain, a light appeared far off in the East. As it came closer to him, it became brighter. He became frightened and wanted to run. However, he heard an inner voice say, 'You have searched for twenty-one years. You have fasted and meditated for twenty-one days. You have prayed for enlightenment and confirmation, and you want to run away now?' And so Dr Usui quietened his intellect and said to himself, 'No, if the light is for me, I accept the enlightenment.' The light became very bright and streamed across the heavens to illuminate his third eye. Dr Usui felt he had died and gone to heaven, because he had never been in such a euphoric state. His entire field of vision was a rainbow of colour. Bubbles of gold, white, blue and violet came out of the rainbow. Each bubble contained holographic Sanskrit characters that he had discovered in the writings of the Tibetan Buddhist teachings. A voice said, 'These are the keys to healing: learn them; do not forget them; and do not allow them to be lost.'

Dr Usui saw and heard, until eventually he heard himself proclaim in his own mind, 'I have them; I will not forget them; and I will not allow them to be lost.' Then he awakened to find himself still on this earth. He quickly gathered his thoughts and his few belongings and began his walk down the mountain. He was excited! He was energized! He wanted to get back to the monk to tell him of the experience. This was the first miracle of the morning.

The second miracle occurred when, in his haste, Dr Usui stubbed his toe. He reached down to check the bleeding and to comfort his pain and, as he did so, realized that both the pain and the bleeding had stopped very quickly. Something was very different about the energy in his hands. They were very hot. Dr Usui healed his toe and continued his journey down the mountain. When he became hungry he stopped at a home that served travellers. He ordered cold rice and cold tea. In a few moments, a girl with a bandage wrapped around her head and jaw brought Dr Usui his meal. He asked the girl what was wrong. She told him she had a toothache. Encouraged by his own healing, he offered to heal the girl. She was in great pain and accepted his offer gladly. Dr Usui put his hands on the girl's jaw and head. Within a few minutes the pain and swelling were starting to disappear. When Dr Usui had finished his meal he went to pay the *papa san*, but the *papa san* said, 'Thank you, sir monk, but I cannot accept the money. You have rendered unto my daughter a service for which I do not have the money to pay. Please accept the food in exchange for the healing services you have rendered.' Dr Usui accepted the food in exchange for his services as a healing instrument. The third miracle was manifest.

The fourth miracle occurred when Dr Usui arrived in Tokyo the next day and went to tell the Zen monk all that had happened. He found the monk in great pain from his arthritis. While he shared his experience he placed his hands on the monk and very quickly the pain disappeared. The old monk was truly amazed. Dr Usui asked the monk for advice on what to do with the keys and the energy healing he had received. He wanted to learn more about its use and how to develop it. The monk told him to meditate. In his meditation he was directed to go to the 'beggar kingdom' in Tokyo. This place was controlled by a beggar king who had a fiefdom of beggars. Dr Usui sought out the beggar king and asked if he could work with the infirm and afflicted. The king admitted him, but did not think he would be successful.

Dr Usui was very disciplined and dedicated. For seven years, he gave Reiki energy, from early morning until late at night. He worked with young and old. Many beautiful results occurred during this time. However, one afternoon he took a walk to the edge of the beggar kingdom where he saw a young beggar who looked very familiar. Finally, Dr Usui asked the beggar if he knew him and and the beggar answered, 'Of course I know you. Do you not remember me? I am one of the first beggars you ever treated.' Dr Usui said 'I treated you and you are still a beggar?' The beggar looked at him and said, 'Oh, Dr Usui, yes. I did just what you told me. I went to the temple to get a name, and went out into society. I even got a job and married, but soon the responsibility became too great. I decided I would rather be a beggar. Then I wouldn't even have to be responsible for myself.' At that moment, Dr Usui realized the importance of an exchange of energy. People needed to give back for what they received – that way life would not be devoid of value. Dr Usui turned around without finishing the conversation and went to his room. He collected his few belongings and left the beggar kingdom. As he was returning to the monastery, he was greeted in spirit by the teachers who had greeted him on Kuri Yama. They gifted him with very important elements: the healing of the spirit, and the understanding of the responsibility of the recipient in the total healing process. Dr Usui realized that he had done the reverse of the Buddhists in concentrating on healing the body and not the spirit. He was then given the Five Spiritual Principles of Reiki by the teachers (see p. 17 for the Principles set out in full).

The Five Spiritual Principles created significant changes in the subsequent works of Dr Usui. He learned that he had been giving away, without requiring the recipient to take any responsibility for the process, and that there had not been an exchange of energy for the services rendered.

The new teaching called for spiritual concepts to be integrated with the physical aspect of the Reiki energy.

Dr Usui realized that living these Spiritual Principles would effect changes in his own life and in the healing he administered to others. He observed how his auric field radiated the Principles into the etheric field of the recipient, altering the recipient's consciousness and equally affecting the healing that was taking place. He also learned that, as the Reiki instrument grew through applying the Spiritual Principles on a day-to-day basis, the essence was manifested on all levels of the person's life. The way in which they acted, reacted, understood and provided advice to themselves and others was changed from the 'I-Ego-Power' of man, to the divine will of the 'I AM' consciousness of God.

Reiki is from the heart. It is only through the heart that the fullness of life can be known. The heart is the doorway to Love: love of self, of Christ and of God within, and the outpouring of divine love in God's creation. From the abundance of God-fulfilling love present, we can love our fellow brothers and sisters and come to know the true meaning of unconditional love.

Dr Usui continued to teach Reiki throughout the islands of Japan until his transition in about 1926. Between the years 1900 and 1926, he gathered a following of sixteen teachers. One of these was Dr Chujiro Hayashi, whom he asked to ensure that the teachings be preserved. Dr Hayashi founded the first Reiki clinic, in Tokyo. In the years preceding the Second World War, he decided to train two women in order that Reiki should survive the war, because he knew that many men would die. His inner vision, having prescience of the war, guided him in this action. One of the women, Hawayo Takata, was born on the island of Hawaii in 1900. She was the child of Japanese parents, but a citizen of the USA. In 1935 she was a widow with two small children and was at the end of her physical strength. She was suffering from a number of chronic illnesses and was guided to go to Japan to seek help with her health. She went to traditional doctors for treatment. As she was lying on the operating table waiting to have an operation, she had a strong feeling that the operation was unnecessary. She spoke to the doctor about it and asked him if there was another form of treatment which could be used. He suggested that she go to Dr Hayashi's Reiki clinic. She began daily treatments with two channels of Reiki, and after a few months her complete health had returned. She became one of the two women that Dr Hayashi decided to train and, after a year in Japan, she went back to Hawaii to live with her daughters. Dr Hayashi visited her in Hawaii in 1938 and made her a Reiki Master. In 1941 she succeeded him as the Grand Master and continued to work in Hawaii for many years. When she was in her seventies she began to train Reiki Masters. On 11 December 1980 she passed away, leaving 22 Reiki Masters in the USA and Canada. In August 1980, shortly before she died, Hawayo Takata and some of the Reiki Masters founded the American Reiki Association, which was to organize the passing on of the knowledge of Reiki.

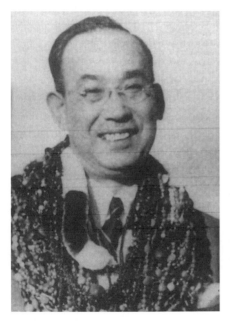 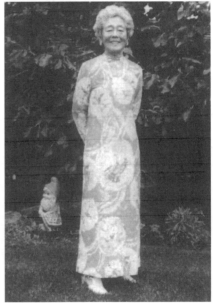

Figure 7: Dr Churijo Hayashi.   Figure 8: Hawayo Takata.

Today, Reiki is represented by three organizations which have succeeded the first. Two are based in the USA and the third in Europe. One is called The American International Association of Reiki; another The Reiki Alliance; and the third is The International Association of Reiki, which has offices in Scotland, Poland and the Czech Republic. At present, there are over 600 Reiki Masters in the world. The Reiki message continues to be spread by those who are dedicated to its principles.

Many Reiki Masters have augmented the method of Reiki by adding their own areas of specialization to the basic technique. They hope to enrich the training of the student by including other metaphysical, esoteric, spiritual and holistic teachings. We should remember that the healing draws on the infinite resources of God. Mankind is the co-operative instrument of the Universe, through which God channels the divine inspiration for peace and wholeness.

Ultimately, health begins with the spiritual aspect of man being awakened to the unconditional love of God. This awakened man then takes full responsibility for his choices in life and is empowered for his own healing. This is the aim of the teachings of Dr Usui, and certainly is also my aim.

Chapter 2
The Five Spiritual Principles of Reiki

Just for today, I will let go of anger.
Just for today, I will let go of worry.
Today, I will count my many blessings.
Today, I will do my work honestly.
Today, I will be kind to every living creature.

Dr Mikao Usui

Just for Today, I Will Let Go of Anger.

To let go of anger is to release what is blocking us from loving unconditionally. Anger is really an unnecessary emotion, which separates us
from the Universal Consciousness. When our expectations about ourselves and others get the best of us, when we or they fail to satisfy these
expectations, or our needs and desires, then we become angry. The people we are angry at have no realization of our anger. Most of the time, it
hurts us more than it could ever hurt them. Remember that all beings are
brought into our lives as a mirror, and are the direct reflection of the
cause and effect created by ourselves. Through the people we bring into
our lives, our mirrors, we can discover the weak points in our egos. To be
angry is very destructive of our inner harmony. Be aware of what causes
the anger – just what is the expectation and/or demand? Feel the emotion fully and release it. Anger is a reaction; the response is love.

Do not blame others by pointing out their faults.
You will find upon self-examination
that the faults you see in others are in you.
When you correct yourself, the world becomes correct.
Sai Baba

Just for Today, I Will Let Go of Worry.

When we worry, we have forgotten that there is a divine purpose in everything. When we are aware that we have lived each day the best we can, we know that the rest is up to the Universe. When we worry, we separate ourselves from the Universal wholeness. Also, we are not trusting that all is in divine order. To worry creates more limitations. Surrender to the plan of our higher self. All is in divine order. Release and trust.

Nothing is cast away by the mind. As
a consequence, grief, worry and misery
continue to simmer in it.
If only the mind can be taught renunciation,
one can become a spiritually serene person.
Sai Baba

Today, I Will Count My Many Blessings.

Counting our blessings means to be grateful for all of the abundance in our lives. We are thankful not only for what we have received, but also for what we know and trust will be provided. As we acknowledge and give thanks for our every blessing, large and small, we attract more blessings to us. Our fear of not having (lack) keeps us from accepting what is truly ours by divine right. What we are able to see, we shall have; what we think, we shall create. If we feel subconsciously unworthy of receiving abundance or blessings from the Universe, we will in some way block the flow of life's riches and blessings to us. Riches not only in a material sense, but also riches emotionally, mentally and spiritually as well. I see how abundantly I am blessed in my life. All things nourish me and I am grateful.

To those who have an insight into life,
everything has meaning.
To those
whose eyes are open,
everything fits into place.
Sai Baba

Today, I Will Do My Work Honestly.

To live life honestly is to be aligned with our higher self's purpose. By being honest with ourselves and facing the truth in all matters, we can live a truly harmonious life. Truth brings clarity. When we are honest with ourselves, we project honesty onto others. By being honest in our work, this truth is reinforced by the resulting love for ourselves and others. This honesty creates harmony in our lives and in our world. We complete the task with less effort. As we clearly see and acknowledge the lessons, our life opens before us.

Truth is your Father
Love is your Mother
Wisdom your son
Peace is your daughter
Devotion is your brother
and spiritual seekers
are your friends.
Sai Baba

Today, I Will Be Kind to Every Living Creature.

As we love and are kind to all living creatures, we experience a sense of unity. We are all of one source. By not being kind to someone we are not actually loving and respecting ourselves, for we are a part of one another. When we accept all aspects of ourselves, then we can accept others. It is always from ourselves to others, from others to ourselves. We are reflections of the divine light. Kindness is love.

19

Do not do unto another
what you *do not like*
to be done unto yourself.

For the other is you.

Sai Baba

Chapter 3
Degrees and Initiations

There are four degrees of Reiki.

The First Degree

In the first degree, four of your energy centres are reawakened and attuned. The energy centres are known as chakras. At this first level your visionary qualities can become more open, which will help you to experience your soul, that eternal light, and its purpose. You are permanently aligned with love. The first degree attunements are primarily focused on the physical body, so that it can respond by opening up to accept and transfer greater quantities of the life force energy. The attunements will raise the vibratory level of the four spiritual centres:

1) The initiation of the heart centre awakens you to unconditional love and attunes both the physical heart and the thymus, our 'spiritual heart', as well as attuning the heart chakra on the etheric level.
2) The initiation of the throat centre awakens the inner being to the aspect of trust and communication. It attunes the thyroid gland and, on the etheric level, the throat chakra.
3) The initiation of the third eye centre awakens the potential for intuition, a deeper knowing and connection to the divine will of this Universal energy that is Reiki. The attunement is on the pituitary gland, which is our centre of intuition and higher consciousness, and the hypothalamus which controls the body's temperature and our moods. The attunement on the etheric level is of the third eye chakra.

4) The initiation of the crown centre aligns you to this higher form of energy, and to spiritual consciousness. It attunes the pineal gland, which is sometimes known as 'the receiver of the light', and attunes the crown chakra on the etheric level.

The Second Degree

In the second degree, you learn absent healing. Reiki Two energy works very deeply on the mental and emotional causes of dis-ease. The second degree places great emphasis on adjusting the etheric rather than the physical body which is the focus of Reiki One. It tends to stimulate the intuitive centre that is located at the pituitary gland – the body's 'telepathic centre'. After the second degree initiation, this centre seems to become sharper and more focused and, as a result of this process, the Reiki Two students often find themselves more aligned to their Higher Selves.

The Third Degree

In the third degree, the lower energy centres are opened and attuned. This is the first step to becoming a Reiki Master. You begin an apprenticeship programme with a Reiki Master which lasts about two years. The student must be so aligned with the system of Reiki that there is no doubt in their whole being that it is their sole purpose and destiny to become a Master.

Everything you do, everything you say, is an example and demonstration of Reiki. You are living your Reiki. You are Reiki!

The Fourth Degree

In the fourth degree, you are initiated as a Reiki Master. Not many people take this path, but once they do, it is a pathway filled with growth and blessings. The fee for the Reiki Master's degree is very high, and it is this fee which provides a large obstacle to overcome. It proves the worth of the Fourth Degree to the one aspiring to become a Master.

I have never regretted my choice to become a Master and have been blessed in my life of service and dedication with the use of Reiki.

Reiki Is in Us

I believe that Reiki is inherent in all beings. It is something we are born with, which lies dormant within us until it is awakened by a Reiki Master. During the initiation process, an inner healing aspect is reawakened within us, so that we are attuned to the energy of Reiki.

Each person's experience with the initiation is different, because we are all unique individuals. Many people find the experience deeply moving. In some way, their lives are changed and they are never the same afterwards.

'Where love is, great changes and healing take place.'
Mari Hall

Come and Walk beside Me

Many students tend to put their teachers on some sort of pedestal, as if they were a guru and had all the answers. This truly disempowers the student and gives false power to the teacher. This is what I say to my students: 'I am not a guru, nor do I have your answers. You are your own best teacher. I merely walk beside you as a loving sister encouraging the steps you take on your journey. As I teach you, you are teaching me.'

It is my hope, should you choose to take this path, that you find a person who is happy to walk beside you as you start your journey with this wonderful form of natural healing.

'You are your own best guru, your own best teacher. The answers are always inside you.'
Sai Baba

Treating Yourself

Treating yourself with Reiki is so simple. Everywhere you are, Reiki is. Whenever you feel stress or pain, or are feeling generally 'out of sorts', all you need to do is give yourself a treatment by placing your hands on yourself.

The daily use of Reiki brings about an inner balance, so that many illnesses will not be able to develop. Your emotions will be balanced. Your life indeed takes on a new quality and peace. When you are using Reiki, you are loving yourself and the creative force within you. This loving energy helps you to transform your will and ego to 'Thy-will-be-done'. The use of Reiki in our personal lives offers us a means of balance, so that we attain a healthy mind, body and spirit. Reiki helps you to experience self-love directly and, as a result, you develop a loving relationship with yourself.

A Suggestion for Daily Self-Treatments

Reiki does not end after you take the seminar. Each person must take on the responsibility of treating themselves. Only you can determine your rate of progress, by the level of commitment you are willing to make. You are your own master and being committed to your own self-healing is the best present you can give yourself.

Lie down or sit comfortably. Start with your head and slowly work down over your whole body, front and back. Include all your chakras, organs, even the soles of your feet. Allow your intuition to guide you to the areas that you feel need energy. This is excellent to do when you first wake up in the morning, or when you are going to bed.

Many people first take a Reiki course in order to bring about a sense of well-being in themselves. Once this is realized, then it is natural to turn it outwards to others.

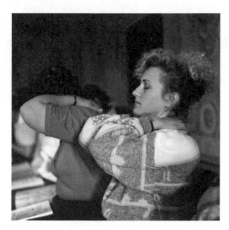

Figure 9

Treating Others

During the first degree course, you will be taught several positions to use in the treatment of other people. These are only suggestions, but they are positions I have found effective. I advise you to allow your hands to go intuitively where they want to during a treatment.

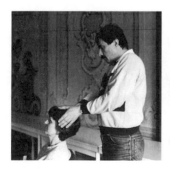

Figure 10

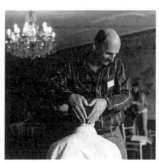

Figure 11

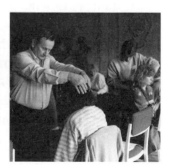

Figure 12

Chapter 4

Suggested Steps and General Principles for Working with Reiki

The Setting for Treatment

Reiki works on a busy street, a train, or anywhere. However, I have found it best to have a specific room or area where you work which is harmonious. It is very relaxing for the person who receives the energy, and at the same time helps you to be relaxed and open.

Work Space and Comfort

It is best to have a massage table that is the proper height for you to sit at during treatment. This table will provide comfort both for the person receiving the energy and yourself, as you are both supported. It is important because the treatment may last an hour.

If a massage table is not available, you could use a dining table, with a foam pad on it, or blankets to pad the space where the person will lie. If the person is bed-ridden, position yourself so that you can easily reach them without discomfort. It is less tiring to keep your own back straight than to be bending over or standing for long periods of time. Remember that comfort for both of you is important.

Clothing and Covering of the Recipient during Treatment

The person remains clothed during the treatment. If they have tight belts, they can be loosened. Shoes can be removed, as well as any binding outer garments.

During the session, be sure to provide the recipient with adequate cover so that they remain warm. Remember that Reiki radiates heat, and when the hands change location, a cooling can take place. If the room is cool, it could be chilling to the person, so you might cover them with a lightweight blanket. This can also be the case in the summer months.

Hygiene

It is important for you to know that your hands are not magnets for negative energy. They do not collect energy, but rather balance and harmonize everything that they touch. Certainly wash your hands before and after a treatment, where it is possible. If you are treating an open infection, wear protective sterile gloves or place a sterile gauze bandage over the infected area, before putting your hand down. Keep the treatment area in a state of cleanliness and order.

Music and Being Centred

Meditative music is very conducive to the relaxation of the recipient and the channel alike. It is most important that you are in a state of harmony. If you are 'centred', then a greater quality of energy can flow through you. Stress = disharmony; relaxation = harmony. If you are in a state of disharmony, work on yourself first. This demonstrates your willingness to apply the principles of Reiki to yourself, and enables you to become balanced and open before you begin working with another person. If you are in a relaxed state, the other person will relax much more readily.

Invocation before Treatment

Although no invocation is required to make Reiki work, if you have a religious philosophy you may wish to say a silent prayer before placing your hands on someone, such as:

'Thank you for allowing me to be an instrument for your divine healing energy. May it go to all people who are willing to receive it.'

Before the Treatment

Talk with the person, to find out what the physical and/or emotional imbalances might be. Four sessions are usually required to complete the initial energy balancing. Treat with as many sessions as you both feel are necessary for the healing effect to take place. If it is possible, all four treatments should be given on successive days. This will stimulate the body to cleanse itself of any toxins. I also recommend to people that they drink a lot of water (at least 2 litres every day), to support the natural detoxification process.

Touching: a Professional Attitude

Many people have difficulty touching or being touched in the private reproductive areas of the body. In most cases it is not necessary to make direct contact, thus eliminating any uneasiness.

More about Touching

A big difference between some other forms of energy work and Reiki is that we touch the body. With some other forms of energy work, the therapist works in the aura or person's field of energy. The philosophy is that, if the aura is in a state of harmony, then the physical body will follow. This is true. When we are touching the physical body, the energy is also going into the aura, so that it can become balanced. When you place your hands on someone, they know that you care about them and that you are there for them in that present moment. I believe that we do not touch each other enough. We touch our children, but at some mysterious time, we stop touching them. They are 'too old for a cuddle'. I see various ages and sizes of people, all of whom have an inner child in them who is saying, 'please hug me and love me'. We do not usually ask for a hug, because we are afraid of rejection. Reiki is a way of loving and being loved. We can reach out and touch that inner child which is in all of us, with unconditional love.

Talking during the Treatment

Quiet conversation can be helpful, especially if the recipient feels like opening up and discussing the emotions surrounding the state of their unwellness. However, do not feel it is necessary for them to talk or that you must investigate to find the cause, if the person does not want to share this information. Sometimes, emotional discussions can be inhibiting to the healing process, causing unnecessary tension, pain and remorse. Since Reiki works on all levels of the body, mind and spirit, it is not necessary for you to counsel. By providing Reiki to take away physical pain, the person will, in their own time, go inward and begin to gain awareness of the emotional factors, which may well be the cause or the result of this particular unwellness.

Distracting noise, such as children playing or the television being on, are not conducive to the healing session. If you must be interrupted to have a conversation, it is suggested that you do so out of the healing setting. Use discretion.

Hand Pressure and the Needs of the Recipient

Place your hands on the body using relaxed and gentle touch. Any pressure or heaviness from your hands may be uncomfortable to the recipient. To ensure that your hands are relaxed, you must be comfortable. Reposition yourself if you are straining from the position you are in. If you are uncomfortable, you will think more about your discomfort than the needs of the recipient. The healing setting must include your comfort, except in an emergency, when the other person's needs outweigh your own. 29

It is important to consider the needs of the recipient. There are many variables, due to the differences between the individuals you will treat. The following questions should be asked of all clients:

1) Is the room temperature too warm or too cold? The temperature should be comfortable.
2) Does the client need a pillow under their head, for comfort?
3) Does the client need a pillow under their knees? This can help to reduce the pressure on the lower back, which is especially helpful for people who have lower back problems, including pregnant women and women with a tilted uterus.

You want the recipient to be comfortable at all times in the healing setting. The temperature, lighting, music, and your state of relaxation and harmony all need consideration. Experience will provide you with additional ideas of how best to meet the needs of the recipient. The most important factor is to be loving.

Permission for Treatment and the Exchange of Energy for Your Time (Fee)

Throughout the world, there are different regulations governing the practice of treating people. Obviously, if you are a doctor who is also practising Reiki, you can apply Reiki whenever you want to and feel that it is necessary. The biggest problem is the amount of time you have to spend with a patient in relation to the amount of time necessary for the treatment. Reiki is being used successfully by many different professional groups, such as masseurs, medical assistants, nurses, midwives, drug counsellors, psychotherapists and beauty therapists.

It is very important that you never make a diagnosis, or even use the word 'diagnosis'. Never advise the client to discontinue medication which their doctor has prescribed; nor should you prescribe any medication, unless you are a medical practitioner. Never undertake any action which will invade beneath the skin's surface.

Some people who are doing Reiki as a profession call it a relaxation technique and are able to do this as the person is indeed relaxed. As the client remains dressed, you are not coming into direct contact with them.

Legal regulations vary from country to country. I advise you to find out about the legal requirements of your professional organizations, before using Reiki as part of your work. It is better not to use the term 'patient', but to use the words 'client' or 'recipient' to describe the people you are treating, so that people do not feel you might be illegally running a medical practice. In all cases where you have any doubt, check the legal situation in your country.

When I was working in Great Britain, I joined the National Federation of Spiritual Healers, as this organization is legally recognized in the UK. Doctors even refer people to members of this organization for treatment.

With regard to payment, people are not paying you (giving you an exchange of energy) for the Reiki energy, but rather for your time. You have a worth or value. Giving and receiving should be in balance. There needs to be an exchange either of services, or of money, for this time. Often, when we work with someone in the family, there is a natural exchange taking place, where people are doing things for each other. Reiki practitioners do establish a fee when they offer their time to channel this energy on a professional basis. The fee sets a value on the service: wellness has a value, and ultimately reflects the feeling of worthiness and self-love of the person seeking to change their health.

The person must ask for treatment – this is a spiritual law. By asking, they open themselves to receive and have expressed a conscious decision to be involved in the process. The recipient is the healer. The channel is only an instrument through which the energy flows. If you do not receive permission, or are not asked, and work on someone anyway, you are exerting your will, your ego, on them. This is not Reiki.

Sensitivity to the Recipient's Pain

It is not uncommon to be sensitive to the recipient's pain. Normally, you feel the pain in the same area of your body as the person who is receiving the energy. This does not mean that you are taking on their pain or energy and will keep it. The level of feeling is merely a barometer, telling you how much energy the recipient will need to balance the area where the pain is located.

Reiki is *not* a system of taking on or extracting pain from someone. If you are left with pain once the session is complete, then you have, at some level, desired (consciously or unconsciously) to retain the person's pain. This usually occurs when you have the thought 'I want to make you well', or 'I will heal you and take away your pain'.

In many instances, I find people develop more sensitivity to feeling, the more they use Reiki. You begin to have a sensitivity to the environment, as well as personal energies. When this sensitivity is developed, it leads to the perception level called 'clairsentience' or clear feeling. Clarity comes when a person clearly distinguishes the origin of the energy, and controls the influence it projects.

Learning to know the difference between your feelings, pains and energy balance, from those of another person, takes training. It is best to ask yourself objectively: 'Is this my own emotion, or pain?' Always be aware of how your own body feels before placing your hands on someone else.

Once you have been reawakened by a Reiki Master, when you place your hands on yourself or another person in order to transfer the energy, you may start to feel warmth and/or a tingling sensation. Leave your hands there as long as these sensations remain as intense. Once the feeling starts to dissipate, move your hands to another area. The energy comes through the palms and fingertips of your hands. The registration of your own body subsides, along with the sensation in your hands, when the proper amount of Reiki has been given to the recipient.

Duration and Timing of Treatments

It usually takes about an hour to give a full body treatment. It is always best, if you have the time, to treat the whole body, as you are treating the cause as well as the resulting illness. When you are working on children, it usually takes half of the time, depending on their size. If you are only treating one area of the body, allow 20 to 30 minutes; with children, of course, the time needed will be less.

Healing is a wondrous process. All of us have our own rhythm and time for things. No two people are alike, and because of that uniqueness the experience is quite often different. I find that if I have an expectation of how someone should respond to treatment, I am not being sufficiently open to their healing process. It may appear that one person has immediate relief from their symptoms, while others may experience an aggravation of their symptoms, or the pain may become more intense. In this case it can indicate that the healing is taking place on a deeper level; on a physical level, the acceleration of the healing process can cause an increase in the intensity of the symptoms, which seems quickly to dissipate, usually by the third day. This is referred to as a 'healing crisis'. In such cases giving more Reiki treatments would be indicated.

Daily application of Reiki to yourself and others for 20–30 minutes will help to keep your system balanced, and will act as a preventive against illness and stress.

In the following pages, the specific imbalances are mentioned not for the purposes of diagnosis, they are for your education only. Always trust your intuition when working with Reiki; respond to that inner voice.

Scanning the Body

1) Relax and centre yourself. Take a few deep, relaxing breaths. Stretch your fingers and your arms. Loosen your shoulders.
2) Sensitize your hands by rubbing them together for a few seconds. Stop, then take another breath so that you are not just feeling the heat that you have just generated by the friction.
3) Begin to feel the energy between your own hands, before you try to feel the energy of someone else.
4) Imagine where the edge of the person's aura is, then use your hands as an extension of your mind. It is important to scan for what is there, not what your mind might think is there. This is not a mental exercise,

but a feeling one. Start at the head and move your hands down one side of the body, keeping them in the aura, just above the body's surface.

5) When you reach the feet move up the other side of the body, back towards the head. (It does not matter which side, left or right, you start with, as long as the whole of the body is covered.) Make your movements graceful and keep your fingers moving as they follow the contours of the aura.

6) Make sure that you continue to breathe normally. If you hold your breath, it will keep you from feeling anything.

7) Keep your spine straight, or at least return often to a straight back position, so that you do not lose the nerve impulses and lessen your ability to feel.

8) Notice areas of the body that are cold or extremely hot. These are areas of imbalance and will need Reiki.

9) Trust your intuition: the more you practise feeling the energy with your hands, the more sensitive you will become.

Figures 13 and 14 are for your information. Consider them as a map to help you find a specific part of the body. They are not intended to be used for diagnosis. Remember, Reiki directs itself to the area where it is needed.

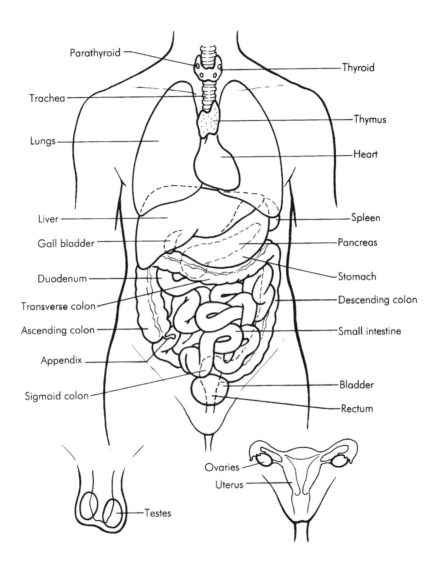

Parathyroid

Trachea

Lungs

Liver

Gall bladder

Duodenum

Transverse colon

Ascending colon

Appendix

Sigmoid colon

Thyroid

Thymus

Heart

Spleen

Pancreas

Stomach

Descending colon

Small intestine

Bladder

Rectum

Ovaries

Uterus

Testes

Figure 13: Trunk of Body with Major Organs – Front View.

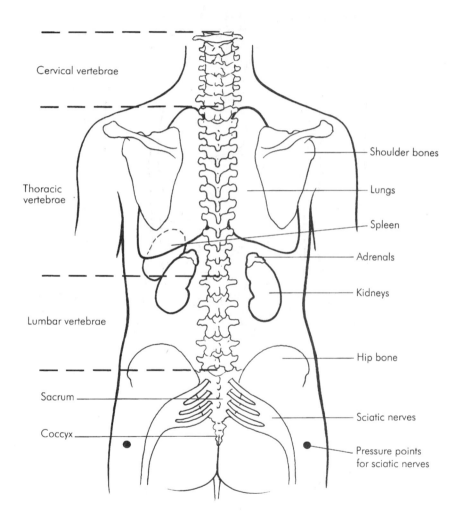

Cervical vertebrae

Shoulder bones

Thoracic
vertebrae

Lungs

Spleen

Adrenals

Kidneys

Lumbar vertebrae

Hip bone

Sacrum

Coccyx

Sciatic nerves

Pressure points
for sciatic nerves

Figure 14: Trunk of Body with Major Organs – Back View.

Chapter 5
Self-Treatment Positions

Front of Head

Position 1

The hands cover the front of the face, with the tips of the fingers touching the forehead (Figure 15). The hands are together, giving yourself space to breathe.

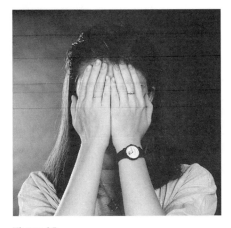

Figure 15

Specific imbalances being treated: sinus blockage; headaches; migraines; strokes; allergies; upper respiratory congestion; hay fever; gum problems; toothache.

Chakra: Third eye
Glands: Pituitary, thalamus

37

Position 2

The tips of the fingers are placed at the midline of the crown of the head. The hands rest gently on the sides of the head (Figure 16).

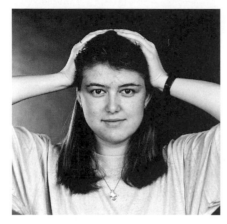

Figure 16

Specific imbalances and functions being treated: mental organization; head injuries; strokes; stress; the left and right hemispheres of the brain; motor and thinking functions; headaches and migraines.

Chakra: Crown

Glands: Pineal, hypothalamus

Back of Head

Position 1

The heels of the hands are cupped at the lower portion of the skull, where the head ends and the neck begins. The fingers extend upward, with the thumbs and index fingers touching (Figure 17).

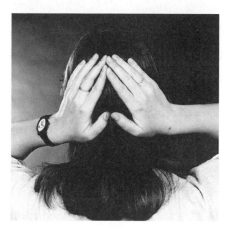

Figure 17

Specific imbalances being treated: headaches and migraines; strokes; eye problems; head injuries; nosebleeds (use with an ice pack applied to the base of the neck).

    Chakra: Third eye

    Gland: Pineal

Position 1 (Alternative)

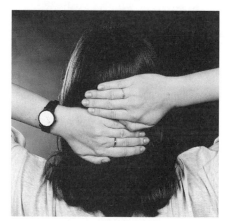

Figure 18

39

This position may be more comfortable. Place hands horizontally behind the head. One hand is on the occipital ridge, the other is below (Figure 18).

See Position 1 for specific imbalances, chakra and gland.

Throat

One hand is placed on the throat and the other rests on the chest, directly below the first (Figure 19).

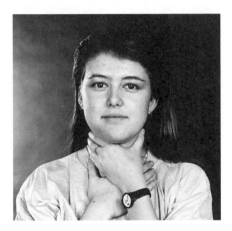

Figure 19

Specific imbalances and functions being treated: energy stimulation; stress; immune system stimulation for better absorption of calcium; nervousness; metabolism problems.

Chakra: Throat

Glands: Thyroid, parathyroid, thymus

Front of the Body

Position 1 (Breast)

Cup the breast, one hand resting on the top of the breast and the other holding the lower part of the breast, so that the entire breast is covered (Figure 20).

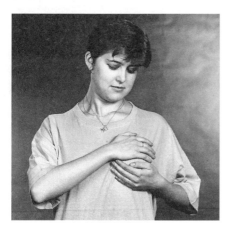

Figure 20

Note: Men also have breasts and will need treatment in this area.

Position 1 (Alternative)

One hand is placed on each breast, the right hand on the right breast and the left hand on the left breast (Figure 21).

Specific imbalances and functions being treated: cysts or tumours in the breast; lymphatic disorders; milk production in nursing mothers.

Chakra: Heart

Glands: Thymus

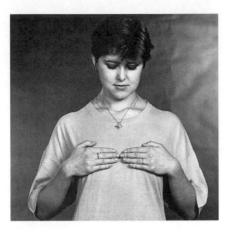

Figure 21

Position 2

Hands are placed under the breast line, with the middle fingertips touching. Hands are placed gently on the body. The fingertips meet at the centreline of the body (Figure 22).

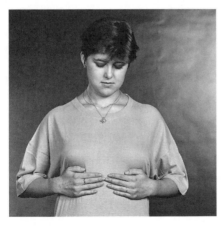

Figure 22

Specific area and imbalances being treated: lymphatic disorders; lungs.

Chakra: Solar plexus

Position 3

Moving your hands down one hand width from Position 2, you should be close to the waistline. Your fingertips are touching and meeting at the centreline of the body (Figure 23).

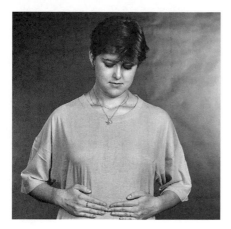

Figure 23

Specific areas and imbalances being treated:

Right side of the body: gall bladder; gallstones; upper colon; colitis; constipation; mucus accumulation.

Left side of the body: upper colon; stomach; ulcers; spasms; digestive problems; pancreas; diabetes; blood sugar imbalance; haemophilia.

Chakra: Solar plexus
Glands: Adrenals

Position 4

Moving your hands down one hand width from Position 3, you should be below the waist, your fingertips touching at the midline of the body (Figure 24).

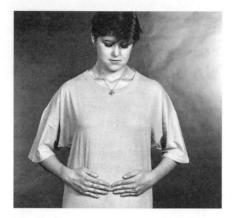

Figure 24

Specific areas and imbalances being treated: lower colon; lower digestive disorders; small intestine; spasms.

Chakras: Sacral and Solar plexus

Glands: Adrenals

Position 5

Your hands point downwards, with the thumbs and index fingers touching. The fingertips touch the pubic bone (Figure 25).

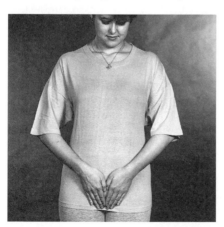

Figure 25

Specific imbalances being treated: female and male reproductive disorders; pain during menstruation; bladder and urinary tract infections; arthritis.

Note: When there is a migraine headache it can be a sign of sexual stress. This position and all three head positions should be used.

Chakras: Root and Sacral

Glands: Testes, ovaries and adrenals

Back of Body

Position 1

Reach up and place the hands on the shoulder muscles. Touch the middle fingers together at the centre of the spine (Figure 26).

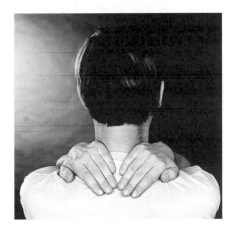

Figure 26

Specific imbalances being treated: tension; throat problems; spinal problems; headaches from neck tension.

Chakra: Throat

Glands: Thyroid and parathyroid

Position 2

These are two separate moves, not to be done at the same time.

A) Take your right hand and reach across the front of the body, placing it on the left shoulder blade, as low as you can comfortably reach (Figure 27).
B) With your left hand reach across the front of your body and place it on the right shoulder blade, as low as you can comfortably reach (Figure 28).

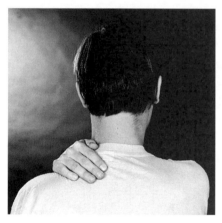 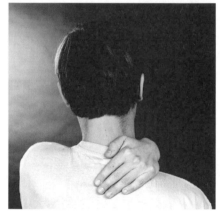

Figure 27   Figure 28

Specific imbalances being treated: nervousness; tension in the upper back; lung and spinal problems.
Chakra: Heart
Gland: Thymus

Position 3

Find your waistline and place your hands with middle fingers touching, one hand higher than the waist (Figure 29).

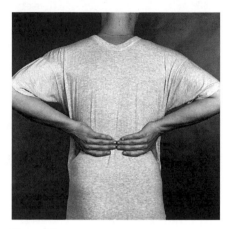

Figure 29

Specific imbalances and areas being treated: diabetes; hypoglycaemia; hyperglycaemia; stress; migraines; kidneys; high blood pressure; infections; adrenal glands; arthritis.

Chakra: Solar plexus

Glands: Adrenals

Position 3 (Alternative)

Place one hand on top of the other over the centre of the spine, at the level of the waist (Figure 30).

See Position 3 (above) for the specific imbalances, chakra and glands being treated.

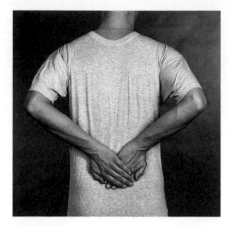

Figure 30

Position 4

The hands point downward, with the heels of your hands at the waistline and the middle fingers touching the top of the tail bone (Figure 31).

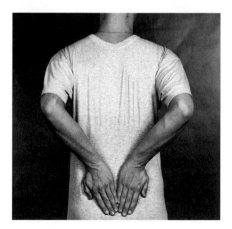

Figure 31

Specific imbalances being treated: intestinal disorders; reproductive disorders; lower back problems.

Chakra: Sacral and root

Glands: Testes or ovaries, and adrenals

Chapter 6
Treating Others

The Best Approach when Working with Someone Else

It is generally best to start at the head, so that the person relaxes. Move around the body, maintaining contact with the person as you change position. When you are finished with the front ask the person to turn over, so that you can work on the back. Again, move around the whole body, so that the entire back, back of the head and back of the legs are treated.

It may be more comfortable for the person to have a pillow under the head when they are lying on their back, as well as a pillow under the knees. When the person turns over onto their stomach, move the pillow under the chest area, so that they can breathe, and the other pillow under their ankles.

If the person has a problem lying on their stomach, if they are pregnant for example, they can lie on one side so that you can treat the back area. Put a pillow between the recipient's thighs in this position to increase their comfort.

Selected positions for the treatment of others are given below. It is best if the person can lie down.

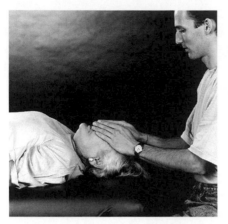

Figure 32: Working at the head.

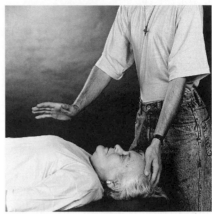

Figure 33: Maintaining contact.

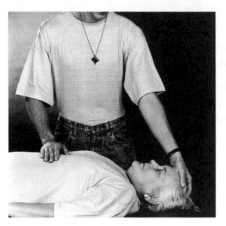

Figure 34: Working from one side.

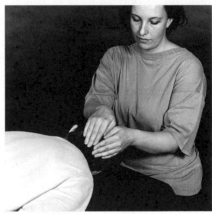

Figure 35: Working on the back of the body.

Head

Position 1

You will be sitting at the head of the person, with the heels of the hands placed on the forehead, index fingers and thumbs adjoining (Figure 36). Gently rest your hands on the person's face, allowing them to breathe easily. You may put a tissue over the eyes if you wish, but do not cover the nose.

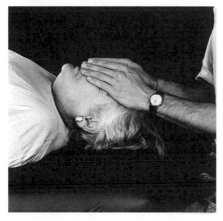

Figure 36

Specific imbalances being treated: eye problems; sinus blockage; headaches; migraines; strokes; allergies; upper respiratory congestion; hay fever; gum problems; toothache.
Chakra: Third Eye
Glands: Pituitary, thalamus

Position 2

Sitting at the head of the person, place the heels of the hand at the centre-line of the crown, your hands extending down the sides of the head towards the ears (as if you are cupping the head in your hands) (Figure 37).

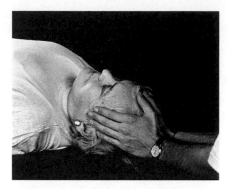

Figure 37

Specific imbalances and functions being treated: mental organization; head injuries; stroke; stress; the right and left hemispheres of the brain; motor and thinking functions; headaches; migraines.

Chakra: Crown

Glands: Pineal and hypothalamus

Back of the head

The person lies on their front, with you sitting at the top of their head. The fingertips touch the lower edge of the skull, where the head ends and the neck begins (the occipital ridge). The hands are joined and placed on the back of the head (Figure 38).

Specific imbalances being treated: headaches; stroke; eye problems; migraines; head injuries; nosebleeds (use an ice pack placed at the back of the neck).

Chakra: Third Eye

Gland: Pineal

Note: Usually this position is done when you are working on the entire back, once the person has turned over.

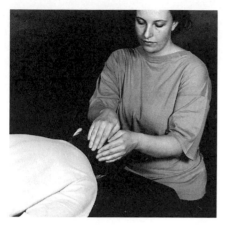

Figure 38

Front of the Body

Position 1

Sitting at the head of the person, bring your hands slightly below the neckline, your index fingers and thumbs adjoining, and rest your hands on the upper chest region (Figure 39).

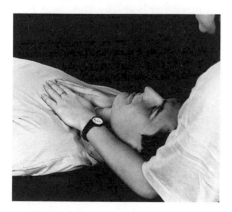

Figure 39

Position 1 (Alternative)

Sitting at the side of the person, put the hand that is the closest to the person on the upper chest region pointing downward towards the lower body. Place the other hand pointing upward on the other side: you will have one hand pointing down and the other pointing up, and it will look as if you are making a semi-circle of energy in the region of the throat and upper chest (Figure 40).

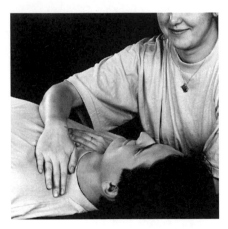

Figure 40

Specific imbalances and functions being treated: energy stimulation; stress; immune system stimulation; weight control; calcium absorption; nervousness; metabolism.

Chakra: Throat

Glands: Thyroid, parathyroid, thymus

Position 2 (Breast)

Treat the breast as needed. Place one hand on one breast and the other hand on the other breast, or you may cup each breast with both hands in turn. If the person does not want their breasts touched, you can work in the aura just above the breast (Figure 41).

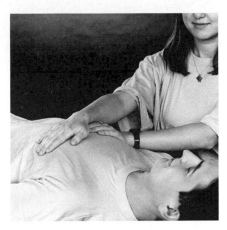

Figure 41

Specific imbalances being treated: cysts; tumours; lymphatic disorders; breast pain during menstruation; migraine headaches where sexual tension is indicated.

Chakra: Heart
Gland: Thymus

Position 3

With hands one hand width lower than the breast, one hand is placed under the breastline on the right side and the other hand is placed on the left side, so that the fingers of one hand touch the heel of the other hand (Figure 42). Rest your hands on the body gently.

Specific areas and imbalances being treated:

Right side: lower lungs; liver disorders; infections; blood sugar imbalances; digestive problems.

Left side: lower lungs; immune system stimulation; spleen; gas release from the heart region.

Chakra: Heart
Glands: Thymus, adrenals

55

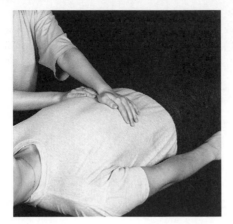

Figure 42

Position 4

Move your hands down one hand width from Position 3. Your hands will be slightly above the waist, the fingertips of one hand touching the heel of the other (Figure 43).

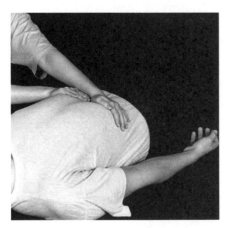

Figure 43

Specific areas and imbalances being treated:
Right side: gall bladder; gallstones; upper colon; colitis; constipation; mucus accumulation.

Left side: upper colon; stomach; ulcers; spasms; digestive problems; pancreas; diabetes; blood sugar imbalance; haemophilia.

Chakra: Solar plexus
Glands: Adrenals

Position 5

Move your hands down one hand width from position 3. Your hands will be below the waist, the fingertips of one hand touching the heel of the other (Figure 44).

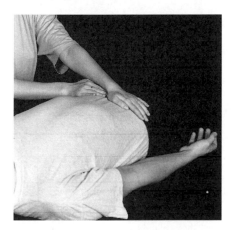

Figure 44

Specific functions and imbalances being treated: colon and upper small intestine; colitis; digestion; constipation; diverticulitis; stress (solar plexus); mucus accumulation; assimilation of nutrients from food.
Chakras: Solar plexus and sacral
Glands: Adrenals

Position 6

One hand is pointing down, resting on the pubic bone to one side. The other hand is pointing up, with the heel of the hand resting on the pubic bone on the other side (Figure 45).

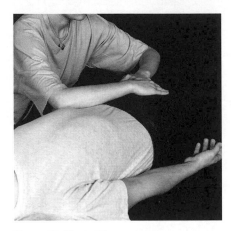

Figure 45: Photo 39

Specific areas and imbalances being treated: lower intestines; colon; bladder; infections; arthritis; cystitis; vagina and uterus; menstrual problems; ovaries; fallopian tubes; migraine headaches where sexual stress is indicated; male reproductive problems.

Note: making contact with the reproductive areas of the body is not necessary if a person is uncomfortable with being touched there. Have your hands just above the area, in the aura: you can rest your arms to support your hands, so that they do not become tired.

Chakras: Root and sacral
Glands: Testes, ovaries and adrenals

Back of the Body

Position 1

Place the heel of one hand on the shoulder muscle, with the middle fin-
gertip touching the channel of the spine (see photo below). The other
hand is placed with the fingertips on the shoulder muscle, and the heel of
the hand touching the channel of the spine (one hand is up and the other
is down) (Figure 46).

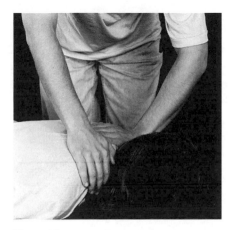

Figure 46

Specific imbalances being treated: tension; throat problems; spinal
problems; headaches from neck tension.
Chakra: Throat
Glands: Thyroid and parathyroid

Position 2

Moving your hands down one hand width, one of your hands is on the
left shoulder blade, the other is on the right shoulder blade and the heel
of one hand is touching the fingertips of the other (Figure 47).

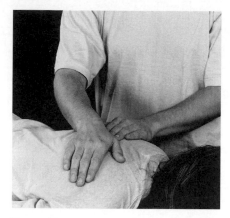

Figure 47

Specific areas and imbalances being treated: nervousness; tension; back of lungs; spinal problems.

Chakra: Heart

Gland: Thymus

Position 3

Move your hands down one hand width from position 2. The heel of your hand is touching the fingertips of the other hand, slightly above the waist. Your hands will be on the adrenal glands and upper portion of the kidney (Figure 48).

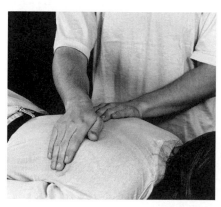

Figure 48

Specific imbalances being treated: diabetes; hypoglycaemia; hypergly-caemia; stress; migraines; infections; spinal problems.

Basically, all body imbalances will require additional treatment time on the adrenal glands. Treating the adrenal glands prevents the person from going into shock, or you can treat the adrenals if they are already in shock.

Chakra: Solar plexus

Glands: Adrenals

Position 4

Move your hands down one hand width. You will be slightly below the waist with the heel of one hand touching the fingertips of the other (Figure 49).

Figure 49

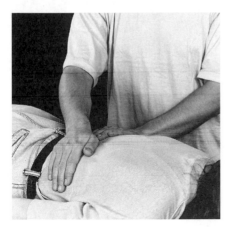

Specific imbalances being treated: kidney problems; arthritis; oedema; high blood pressure; infections.

Chakras: Solar plexus and sacral

Glands: Adrenals

Position 5

One hand is pointing down to the tail-bone and resting on one side of the lower back, to the side of the spine. The other hand is pointing up from the tail-bone on the other side of the lower back, to the other side of the spine (Figure 50).

Specific imbalances being treated: intestinal disorders; lower back problems in the lumbar and sacral areas.

Chakras: Sacral and root

Glands: Testes or ovaries and adrenals

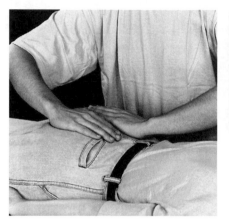
Figure 50

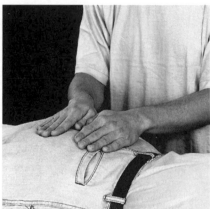
Figure 51

Position 5 (Alternative)

Place one hand horizontally across the lower back. The other hand is placed below it, resting on the spine, across the lower back (Figure 51).

The specific imbalances, chakras and glands being treated are the same as in Position 5.

Feeling the Energy with Your Hands

Once you have been using Reiki for a while you may notice an increase in the sensitivity of your hands. You may start to feel the energy move through the part of the body that you are touching. It will feel like a pulse beat – not the pulse that you feel at the wrist, but a movement of energy. If the area is out of balance you will not feel this at the same time in both hands – it will be erratic. If the area is in balance then the energy will be felt at the same time in both hands – it is synchronized.

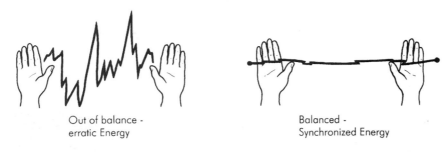

Out of balance -
erratic Energy

Balanced -
Synchronized Energy

Figure 52: Feeling the energy between the hands.

In the following special positions for specific illnesses, I usually wait until I have that feeling of being balanced or synchronized, before I move my hands. I am feeling the energy move, as well as the temperature and/or tingling.

Chapter 7

Special Positions for Specific Imbalances

Earaches, Hearing Loss, Deafness

Place the middle finger gently on the ear opening. The middle finger will be bent to accomplish this. The index finger is placed on the head in front of the ear, while the ring and little finger are placed behind the ear on the head.

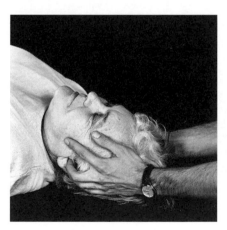

Figure 53: Treating the ears.

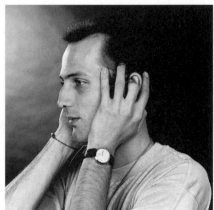

Figure 54: Treating the ears (self).

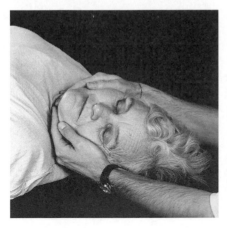

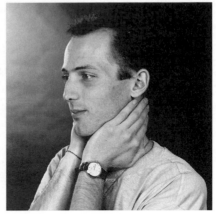

Figure 55: Treating the Eustachian Tubes.

Figure 56: Treating the Eustachian Tubes (self).

Remember to treat under the jaw for earaches, as the Eustachian tubes fill up with pus, fluid and mucus (Figures 55 and 56).

High or Low Blood Pressure Problems, Strokes and Migraine Headaches

Place one hand on the back of the head on one side. The other hand is placed on the neck on the opposite side, over the carotid artery (Figures 57 and 58). Treat until the energy flow is balanced and then place the hands in the reverse positions.

Special notes: In cases of very high blood pressure (over 180), it is suggested that you begin treatment with the hand placed on the neck for only five to ten seconds. Increase the amount of time on the neck each time you work with the person. This precaution will prevent a radical change in the blood pressure, which could cause faintness or nausea. Also, it is important to note that this is not a 'bandage' for blood pressure problems: very often blood pressure problems are a result of other imbalances in the body. It is always best to do a full body treatment.

65

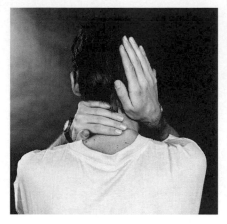

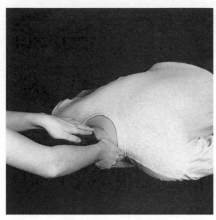

Figure 57: Treating self (treat both sides).   Figure 58: Treating others (treat both sides).

Immune System Stimulation

Place one hand on the thymus gland (medical doctors say this gland is non-functioning). It is a spiritual centre and does take energy. Then place the other hand on the spleen, which is on the left side of your body (Figures 59 and 60). You are balancing the third and fourth chakras together.

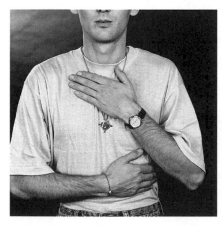

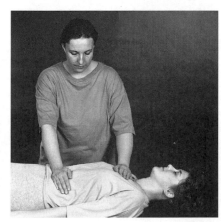

Figure 59: Treating self.   Figure 60: Treating others.

Poor Circulation of the Legs, Varicose Veins and Lower Lymphatic Disorder

Treat the right and left leg alternately. Place one hand at the top of the leg, inside the thigh. The other hand is placed on the groin and the hands touch where the leg and body are joined together (Figures 61 and 62).

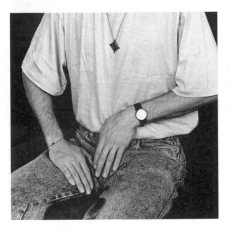

Figure 61: Treating self.

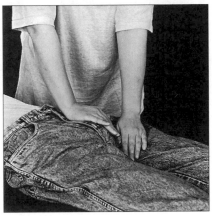

Figure 62: Treating others.

Alternate legs as they become balanced.

Circulation of the Arms and the Lymphatic System

If you are treating yourself, you place one hand under the arm in the armpit, alternating to the other side as you feel the energy becoming balanced (Figure 63).

If you are working with someone else, place your hands under the arm in the armpit, using both hands (Figure 64). This is an excellent position for the treatment of lymphatic disorders, and is a wonderful treatment for toxic build-up in the body. It can also be used for removing cysts in the armpit.

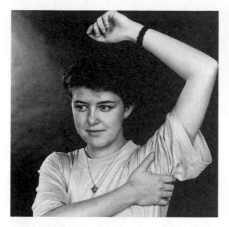

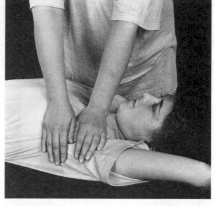

Figure 63: Treating self.

Figure 64: Treating others.

Lung and Related Respiratory Dysfunctions

1) Put one hand down and one hand up on the other's upper chest, as in Position 1 (Alternative) on the front of the body (Figure 65).

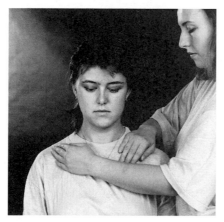

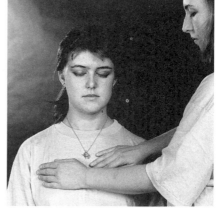

Figure 65

Figure 66

2) The hands are placed on the breastline, as in Position 2 on the front

of the body (Figure 66). Move your hands down one hand width at a

time (Figure 67), leaving your hands in place until there is a dissipation of the energy, and/or you feel the area has come into balance.
Work over the entire lung area; also treat the sides of the body so that
you energize the sides of the lungs. It is easier to treat the side of the
body if the person is lying on their side.

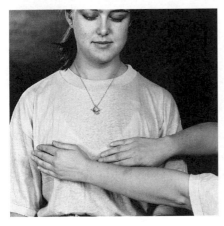 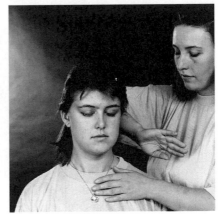

Figure 67   Figure 68

Pay attention to the direction in which your hands are pointing, as you
will need to make a circle with the energy. It does not matter which way
the circle goes. If I started on the right side of the front of the body,
I would work on the back from the left side.

3) On the back of the person, one hand goes up, and the other down, as
   in Position 1 on the back of the body (Figure 69).

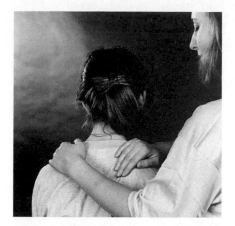

Figure 69

4) Work your way down one hand width at a time, as in Positions 2 and 3 on the back, in order to energize the whole lung area (Figures 70 and 71).

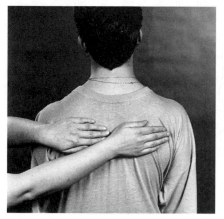

Figure 70

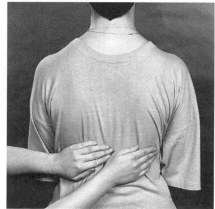

Figure 71

Special note: never place a person who has pneumonia on their stomach. You will have to treat their back by reaching under them, or having them sit up, if possible. Always lie them at a 30 degree angle, to ensure better breathing.

Prostate Problems in Men, and Haemorrhoids in Men and Women

One hand is placed on the lower back in a horizontal position. The other hand is placed over the centre line of the base of the spine, with the fingers pointing down and the middle finger at the very end of the backside (Figure 72). You will be cupping the rear end with your hand.

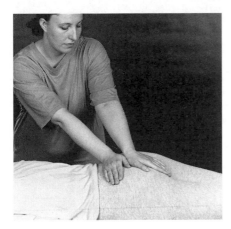

Figure 72

Prevention of Stress

To treat yourself, place one hand over the thyroid gland, at the base of the throat. Place the other hand on the solar plexus (the centre of the body above the navel) (Figure 73).

To treat another person, you follow the same directions as the self-treatment (Figure 74). You should wait until there is a dissipation of energy and/or a feeling of balance.

71

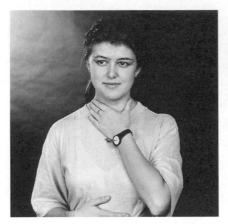

Figure 73: Treating self.

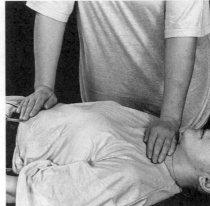

Figure 74: Treating others.

Heart Imbalance and Heart Attacks

1) In the case of all heart imbalance (except heart attack), you must first work under the breast area, as in Position 3 on the front of the body (Figure 75). This position will enable the person to dispel any built up pressure caused by accumulated gas.
2) When the gas is expelled, place your hands directly over the heart in the position shown (Figure 76).

Heart attacks: go directly to the heart. If you know CPR (Cardinal Pulmonary Resuscitation), you would use this technique if the person's heart had stopped beating. If breathing has ceased, then begin resuscitation with one hand on the heart. Reiki has been known to help return a heart to normal operating function after a heart attack (Figure 77).

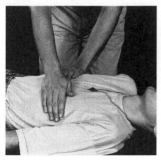

Figure 75

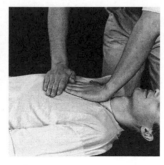

Figure 76

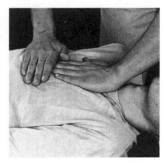

Figure 77

Scoliosis (Hardening and Curvature of the Spine), Arthritis, Whiplash and Related Spinal Injuries

1) Place both hands over the trapezius muscles and leave them there until the energy has dissipated (Figure 78).

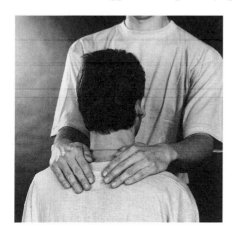

Figure 78

2) Go down the entire back, using Positions 1,2,3 and 4 for treating the back of the body. Move down one hand width at a time so that you cover the entire back (Figures 79–81).

73

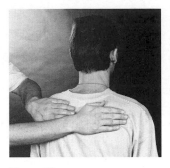
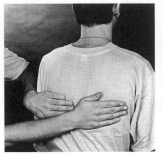
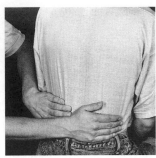

Figure 79   Figure 80   Figure 81

3) Finally, place the hands over the lower back as in Position 5 (Alternative) for the back (Figure 82).

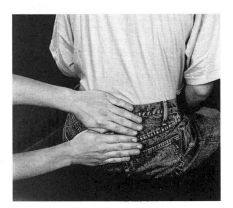

Figure 82

Sciatica

Figure 83 shows a neurological diagram of the sciatic nerve, starting at the sacrum and running down the leg. Note the pressure points on the shoulders and also in the buttocks where there is a dimple. Sciatica should be treated using Reiki in conjunction with chiropractic treatment. Ask the person to get a spinal/sacral adjustment first and give them a Reiki treatment immediately afterwards.

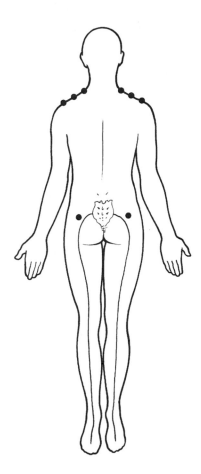

Figure 83: Sciatic nerve and pressure points.

Indicators of pressure points: if they are sore, it is an indication of sciatic problems.

The sciatic nerve starts at the base of the spine and moves down the leg to the bottom of the foot.

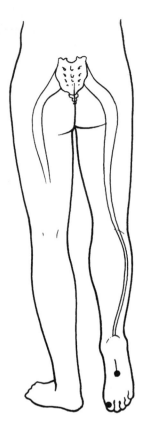

Figure 84: Sciatic nerve.

How to Treat the Sciatic Nerve

1) Place one hand over the sacral bone, with the fingers of the hand pointing down to the tip of the tail-bone. Place the other hand beside it, with the fingers pointing in the opposite direction (Figure 85).

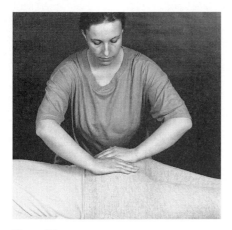

Figure 85

2) Move the second hand down the leg one hand length at a time until you reach the knee (Figures 86 and 87).

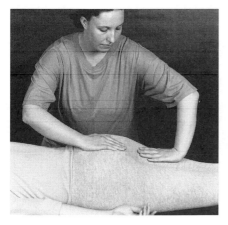 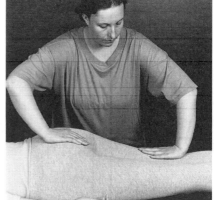

Figure 86   Figure 87

3) Beginning at the knee, place the hands on either side of the leg, so that you are sandwiching the leg between your hands. Work your way down, one hand width at a time, until you have worked on the entire lower leg and sole of the foot (Figures 88 and 89).

77

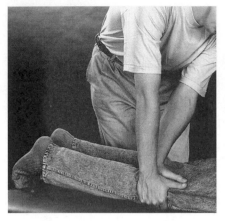

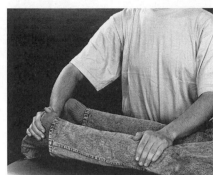

Figure 88   Figure 89

Female and Male Reproductive Disorders; Bladder and Urinary Tract Imbalance

Place one hand over the pubic/uterine area and the other between the legs, with the palm of the hand in front of the reproductive area (Figures 90 and 91). (The recipient is to remain clothed during all treatments.)

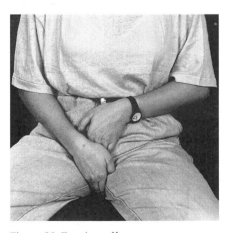

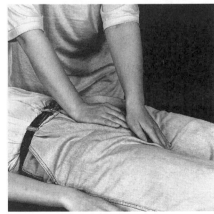

Figure 90: Treating self.   Figure 91: Treating others.

This position can treat the following: yeast infection; herpes; vaginitis; cystitis; urinary tract disorders; testicle infection; low sperm count; and bladder disorders.

To Give First Aid

One hand is placed over the adrenal glands (the glands on top of the kidneys) and the other is placed on the injured area (Figure 92). This is to prevent shock.

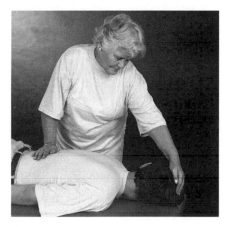

Figure 92

Using Reiki with Acupressure Points

You can use Reiki to activate and balance acupressure points anywhere on the body. The ones shown in Figure 93 are for the sinuses. To activate the acupressure points for the sinus, place the fingertips of one hand on the upper orbital ridge of the eye socket, then place your index finger of your other hand on the centre of your lower orbital socket. For further information about acupressure points consult your library.

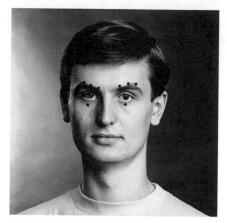

Figure 93

Sandwiching an Area

You can make a sandwich by placing your hands on either side of an area, as indicated in Figure 94. The energy comes from both hands, so that the treatment is intensified. You can sandwich a shoulder, hip, elbow, ankle, hand, or the throat, to name but a few areas. If you are working with broken bones, you can treat through the cast. This is an excellent position for treating wounds, broken bones, damaged muscle tissue and burns.

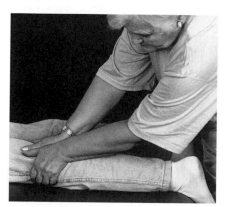

Figure 94

Running Energy through an Area

You can run energy through an arm or leg, or through the soles of the feet or the hands. Leave your hands there until you feel the area become synchronized.

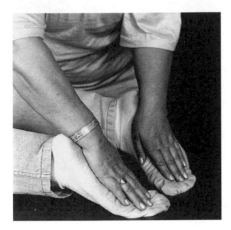

Figure 95: Running energy through the soles of the feet.

Running energy through the arm (Figure 96) can be used to treat the following conditions: arthritis, broken bones, infections, immune system depletion and cancer. Production of white blood cells in the bone marrow is stimulated, which then enter the spleen where they combine with the thymus hormone to produce the 'T'-cell. Running energy through the leg (Figure 97) can be used to treat broken legs and arthritis of the knee, hip or ankle, and to stimulate the immune system.

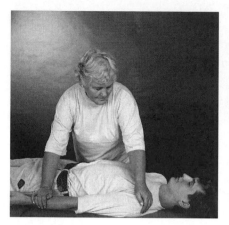

Figure 96

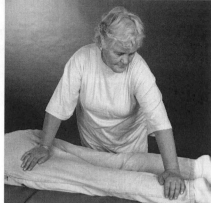

Figure 97

Raising and Lowering Energy

The following are special positions designed to raise and to lower the energy in the body. They should not be done unless it is specifically indicated. To raise the energy in the person's body, place your left hand on their crown and your right hand at the base of their spine (Figure 98).

Specific purposes: increased energy and spinal balancing.

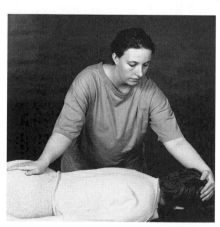

Figure 98

To lower the energy in a person, place the right hand on the top of the head and the left hand at the base of the spine (Figure 99).

Specific purposes: reduces hypertension, excess energy and over-sensitivity.

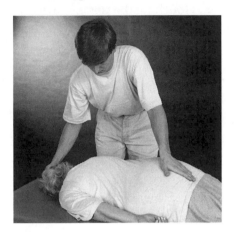

Figure 99

Releasing Spinal Tension

1) Place the thumb and middle finger of the right hand on the occipital ridge at the base of the skull, as indicated in Figure 100, and the left hand at the base of the spine (Figure 101). Wait for the feeling of being synchronized.

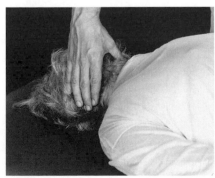

Figure 100

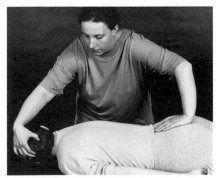

Figure 101

83

2) Move the hands equally towards the centre of the spine, one hand space at a time (Figure 102). Each move is completed when the pulse is synchronized. The hands never lose contact with the body. Slide your hands towards one another, always touching the spine, moving closer to the area of the greatest tension (Figure 103).

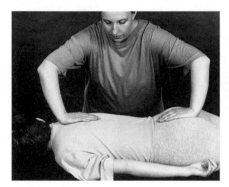

Figure 102

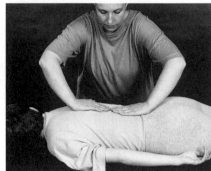

Figure 103

When You Have Finished a Treatment

When you have finished a treatment, in order to ground the energy and discontinue transmission, simply put both hands together, as in Figure 104.

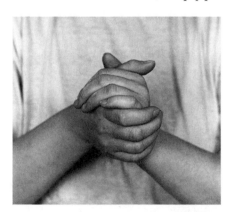

Figure 104

Chapter 8
Other Ways of Using Reiki

Working with a Group of Reiki Instruments

When you begin to work together it is important to be synchronized with one other. This need not take a long time, and is usually accomplished by holding hands, taking a few deep, relaxing breaths and finding your own centre. Once this is done, the energy between each other should feel even. If there are several of you working on one recipient, each person will Reiki a different part of the body. The treatment time will be much less if there are more people working with a recipient. The greatest compliment is when the recipient is so relaxed that they fall asleep.

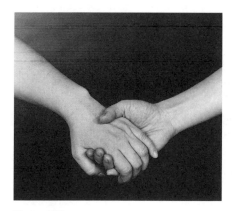

Figure 105

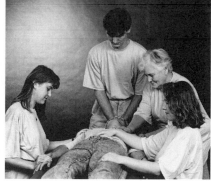

Figure 106

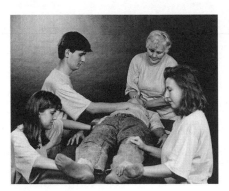

Figure 107

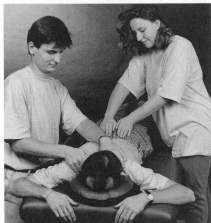

Figure 108

Working Together for the Promotion of Well-being in the New Year

On New Year's Eve 1992, a group of friends, all of whom do Reiki, were together at a lovely chateau in the mountains near Liberec in the Czech Republic. It was close to midnight as we all sat down to meditate and to send energy to the world. It was the end of one year and the beginning of a new one: the country was changing from Czechoslovakia to two separate republics. Using Reiki Two techniques, we directed energy to friends, loved ones and to all people on our planet and to the Universe.

The manager of the chateau asked what Reiki was and whether it could help him. He was suffering from an inflamed shoulder. He had received treatment for it in Russia with some results, but had not found anyone that could help him in the Czech Republic. At first, two of us worked on him twice a day for two days, by the end of which he had gained total relief from the pain. On the last day of our stay, we all sat down and worked on him. As soon as we touched him, he was fast asleep. It was such a peaceful, sweet energy in the restaurant and the start of a happy new year for Jirka!

You can gather a group of Reiki friends and work with each other, or work on someone else. It is a wonderful feeling to use Reiki together in whatever way and, most especially, to send Reiki love all around the world.

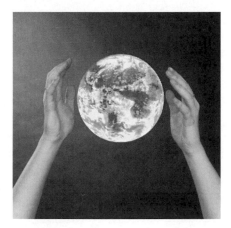

Figure 109

Ways to Connect with Each Other in a Group

When groups of Reiki people come together, we often sit in a circle and put our right hand on the heart of the person on our right (Figure 110); we can also put our left hand over the person whose hand is on our heart. We are feeling the connection of open hearts; the unity and harmony of the entire group. No words are needed: the space is quiet and we are experiencing the never-ending energy of Reiki and our love for one another. We give; we receive; we are one.

Another way to connect is to sit in a long line resting in each other's arms (Figures 111 and 112). We are supported, nourished and loved, as we receive from the person behind us and give to the person in front. It is a beautiful, spiritual experience: a time of togetherness, not separation. We are unified; we are loved, and it is fun.

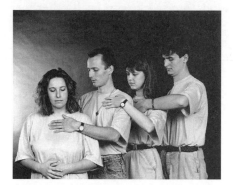

Figure 110

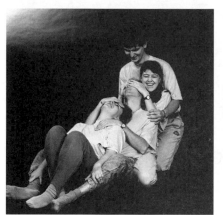

Figure 111

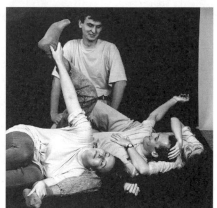

Figure 112

Our Expectations and People's Attachment to Illness

At times, we may expect a particular result when we work on someone else or on ourselves. When that expectation is not fulfilled, we are disappointed. Something else may have taken place, but it was not what we wanted. It is our demand that gets in the way: we must remember that Reiki directs itself, and is perhaps working on a different level from the one we are willing to see. So there may be an internal change, rather than an external one. Do not judge the results of Reiki: it is not your will that will be done. Put your ego aside and be willing to wait for the results to become manifest. Give unconditionally.

Some people are attached to illness on a subconscious level. Even though they say that they want treatment, to give up the illness is a subconscious threat to part of their identity. I have had people come for Reiki treatment with long lists of their diagnoses, starting from the time they were children. 'These are mine', they say. As long as they want to keep them their own on some level, it will be harder to let them go. Reiki Two techniques will help these people to release them. I do encourage people to rid their mind of the concept that they are sick and, rather, to look at the situation as being 'not balanced'. Then we can work together to bring balance about.

> 'Your mind is a truly powerful tool; it creates your reality in every moment. You are as well as you think you are capable of being.'
> Mari

I know you will experience many wonderful results using Reiki. Over the years, I have seen many miracles. I never expect a result; I remain open to what occurs, and I have always been blessed.

Reiki in the Treatment of Babies and Children

Reiki provides the most natural and pleasant way for a mother and father to treat their baby. Parents often hold their baby lovingly anyway, and once one or both of you have learned to give Reiki, you can pass it on to your child every time you stroke or touch it. This energy will intensify the natural relationship that you have with your child. Reiki is a special form of love which all humans thrive on – especially babies.

It is, of course, possible to treat the babies and children of other people, but it is always better for parents to treat their own children, because a loving bond of trust has already been established. I have found that when I treat children, it is best if the child is sleeping, so that he or she is relaxed. I simply sit by their cribs or beds and place my hands on them.

The effects have been quite profound, with some parents finding very relaxed, happy children the next morning and the problems gone or disappearing. It is my recommendation that parents take part in Reiki classes, so that they can treat their own children and support their healing process. This alternative proves to be satisfying in the long run, because it is far less complicated and less expensive.

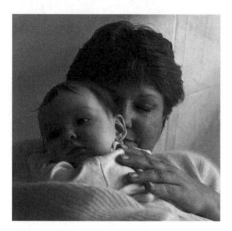

Figure 113

I have some friends who are students of mine in England. I stay with them when I am travelling in the UK. Sometimes, one of the girls will say, 'Mummy, please give me some Reiki – I can't sleep', or 'Can I have some Reiki? – I don't feel well.' I also find their father sitting by their bed, reading a bedtime story, with one hand on his daughter, giving her Reiki. It has become part of their bedtime routine. I am always filled with gratitude to see how Reiki has become so integrated into their lives. The children love it!

Reiki is also excellent for mothers-to-be. When my daughter, Stacey, was expecting my grandson, Jeremy, I gave her weekly Reiki treatments. It was wonderful. The first time I was with her, she put my hand over her womb and said, 'Here is our baby.' She was relaxed and I felt so connected to my family: to my daughter and to the child growing inside her. I was indeed blessed to be able to love into my grandchild throughout his early development and growth. A mother-to-be can also pass

Reiki to her developing baby, influencing the child with that energy for its entire life.

In the Czech Republic there is a hospital for women where all the doctors and nurses give Reiki. In fact mediation music is played in all the labour and delivery rooms. The noticeable results are that the births are easier, mother and child are calm and filled with love, and the connection of the staff with the new families is warm and sincere. A nice way to start a new life, wouldn't you agree?

Treatment of Animals and Plants

Although I have so far discussed using Reiki treatment of oneself and other people, you can also use Reiki to treat animals and plants. Reiki works on all living matter.

When I treat an animal, I notice that it relaxes and tends to be quiet. Cats love to curl up in your lap. They will often push up under your hands to feel the energy. You will soon notice that the Reiki energy flows into animals, just as it does into people. Use your imagination when working with different types of animals. You can put your hands on either side of an aquarium in order to treat fish. I have even worked with a snake – it curled up in my hands! A friend of mine in Scotland developed quite a reputation as a miracle worker. He was called out to look at a friend's horse. The horse was a steeplechase runner which had a lame foreleg and a problem with its shoulder. The vet said that he would have to be put out to pasture, because he would not be able to race again. However, Tom stood on a ladder to treat the horse's shoulder and then worked with its leg. After three treatments, the horse was fine and is still racing! Tom says he likes to work with four-legged animals, as they do not normally answer back. He took me to the stables one day to work with the animals. I was treating a horse when I heard laughter. When I asked what was so funny, I was told that the horse had fallen asleep. I have always said that it is a compliment to the channel when the client falls asleep. This applies to animals too! Another woman that I know treats lambs. The vets call her to come and work with them out in

91

the fields and mountains of Scotland. She is known to be quite a Reiki miracle worker.

I had an opportunity to treat my own dog, Schnapps. He had developed an incurable blood disease. The vet did not give him any hope at all. I took him home from the animal hospital every evening and treated him through the night. I slept with my hands on him. The vet was very surprised that the dog was responding and getting better. When he asked me what I was doing, I explained about Reiki. The vet took the Reiki course and is using it on his 'clients' successfully.

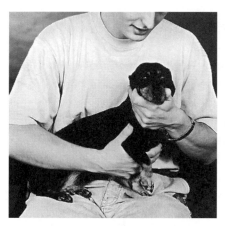

Figure 114

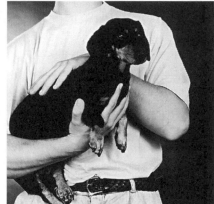

Figure 115

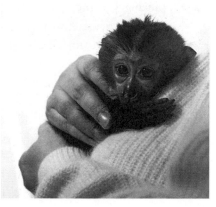

Figure 116

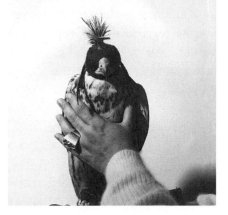

Figure 117

When using Reiki on plants, you can hold the pot in which they are planted between your hands. Hold seeds before you plant them in the ground and use Reiki to energize the water that you use to water them. I am always impressed at how strong and healthy plants are as a result of the treatments. When I am in nature, I hug trees and give them Reiki – but don't be surprised when the tree gives you back energy in return. There seems to be a giving and receiving when working with trees.

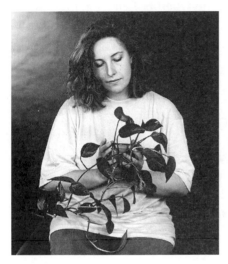

Figure 118

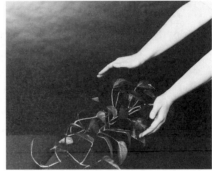

Figure 119

Above all, let your mind be free when you work with animals and plants: follow your intuition. Reiki is unlimited, with boundless energy going to all living matter. Reach out and touch – I promise that you will be pleasantly surprised!

Using Reiki with Death and Dying

I personally think that death is a part of transition, part of the never-ending cycle of rest and activity. We certainly have experiences of letting go in different ways. I have been honoured to be with people, loved ones, as they let go of the physical body, releasing the pain and struggle. They

93

are at peace and filled with the loving energy of Reiki. It is a deeply moving experience for me. It seems as if they are more aware of themselves, the inner light within them, and are secure. Reiki is a gentle and effective means of supporting our loved ones, friends, and even animals, as they pass through this state of transition. Reiki can also be used to treat the family and friends through their grief process. It helps them to let go fully, with love.

Never doubt for a moment, or question whether Reiki is appropriate at this time. It is always the right time to reach out and touch, in all cases. You will be touched as well, by the love and gratitude you experience as an instrument of Reiki.

Absent Healing with Second Degree Reiki

Many people are surprised when they learn that Reiki can be sent to other people over long distances. It can hardly be surprising, once we realize that our bodies can act as receivers, just as a radio or television does for waves sent through the air. We are essentially wireless forms of transmission and receiving.

Natural laws exist which enable us to transfer life energy over long distances. The Reiki method of absent healing is based on these laws, and the key to them can be learned in the second degree of Reiki. It is not necessary to know all the natural laws in order to make use of this technique.

Absent healing is used when it is physically impossible to be with the person needing treatment. It is also a method which can be put to use immediately when you are asked to give treatment to someone. It can certainly be utilized to give additional treatment to a person you are working with in person. You can send them a nightly treatment to support them until you are together again.

If a person has never experienced Reiki, there may be a certain scepticism about the effect of this treatment.

My first experience in doing a treatment in this way was when I was taught absent healing by my Reiki Master. I worked on my daughter who, at the time, was many thousands of miles away, in Hawaii. I could find the various places of her body which needed treatment. I felt her presence with me during the entire time. Two days later, she telephoned and in the course of the conversation told me that she had been relieved of a headache and bad stomach-ache at the very time I had worked on her.

Quite recently, I was teaching in the Netherlands. During the seminar, I felt so lovingly supported and had a sense of warmth flooding my body. I later learned that a Reiki support group made up of my students from Scotland had sent me absent healing at that same moment. Absent healing is indeed powerful and beautiful both for the therapist and the receiver – in this case, I was both.

Many times during second degree Reiki courses, I have asked my students to work on the planet Earth, or on a particular country in need of healing. It always fills us with love and gratitude that we can help our city, state, country and world with Reiki energy.

You should never treat a person by absent methods against their will. Everyone has the right to be healthy or unhealthy. It is best for the person needing the treatment to ask for it. If I am treating a person over a long time, I will ask for a photograph to work with, as well as their full name. I generally do absent healing in the evening, before I go to sleep. I find it a beautiful way to relax.

Mental/Emotional Release Technique with Second Degree Reiki

We often react to negative experiences in our lives in such a manner that it programmes our minds to attract these stressful experiences into our lives time and time again. It makes us painfully right about our belief system. This reaction can also be the cause of our attachment to our resulting illness.

The mental/emotional release technique which is taught in the second degree of Reiki, will enable you to release those attachments to that programmed part of you or another person, enabling the reactive energy to be set free.

Since most physical illness is derived from emotional/mental/spiritual disharmony, this method can be used for all disturbances and imbalances.

The instrument has a great deal of responsibility regarding the use of this technique: it should only be carried out with the full permission of the recipient, and you must take care not to project any judgements onto the person.

When I first went through this process, I released my attachment to someone who was no longer in my life. It was a profound experience. As a result of that experience, I felt able to move forward as 'Mari', unattached. I no longer felt incomplete without that person. This was a major turning point in my life.

One of my translators for the courses in the Czech Republic said that it seemed too easy to work. Yet as the days went by, she noticed that the fear she had when encountering large groups of people had disappeared. This is what she had worked on removing. She is now quite comfortable with large groups, and her personality has changed as she gains in self-confidence.

Reaction is turned into response. As we respond to life, we are able to be objective and go with the flow, rather than being in that reactive and subjective state where we experience being stuck in a situation.

We are free!

Chapter 9

Using Reiki with Other Healing Techniques

Reiki supports and increases the effectiveness of every form of treatment that I know of. Many people combine their existing knowledge and training with Reiki: medical doctors, physiotherapists, psychotherapists, chiropractors and masseurs. People use Reiki with acupuncture, acupressure, colour therapy, crystal healing, homeopathy, breath work, bioenergetics and mind-directed energy.

I myself have used Reiki with several other healing techniques that I have learned, with successful results. Recently, I have studied with a Polish healer in his country. He has people coming to him from all over the world. He taught me mind-directed healing methods. We can see how this energy and the energy of Reiki come together, increasing the effectiveness of both. We worked with people together, and the recipients reported to me their experiences with the combined energy. I have been very fortunate to have had this experience.

Reiki is always the basis. Do not be afraid to experiment with ways in which Reiki can enhance whatever other form of treatment you use, or that you are studying. Reiki is yours to use and will become unique to you as the instrument, as it is combined with whatever other techniques you use, enhancing your work and yourself.

There are many types of harmonizing techniques. In this chapter, I shall deal with a few of them and the ways in which Reiki can be integrated with them to promote harmony. In no way do I claim to be an authority on these techniques, but I have found their use beneficial to my Reiki work.

Reiki with Sound (Toning)

Sound is vibration and our bodies react and respond to different frequencies, or tones. People have their own unique vibrational or base tone, as well as a tone in each of the chakras. We are surrounded by sound: some sounds support us, others sounds can cause us to create imbalance. Sound has been used for healing for centuries by people from various traditions and cultures. Many contemporary healers use toning to alter the energetic field of their clients to improve harmony and health. Different tones and tone combinations can be used for different purposes, such as loosening energy blocks and charging the aura of the body and the chakras. You can, as you are transmitting Reiki energy, also tone into the chakra to increase the energy flow and increase the harmonizing effect. Generally, you can work with a scale of G, as it is the tone that resonates with the earth.

Below is a guideline for the notes of the musical scale to be used with each chakra, and also the colour vibration that is produced with each note. To harmonize each chakra, always trust our intuition about which note to use.

Chakra		Colour	Tone
7th	crown	white	G
6th	third eye	purple	D
5th	throat	blue	A
4th	heart	green	G
3rd	solar plexus	yellow	F
2nd	sacral	orange	D
1st	root	red	G (below C)

Colour Therapy with Reiki

Every colour has its own vibration. Colour is essential to health and we are often attracted to the colours we need to promote balance. Surely, every disease is associated with dysfunction in the chakras. Chakras can be nourished with the colours in which they are lacking. A chakra can be energized with the required colour and the effect increased with Reiki energy. Because every colour has a different vibration, we will have a different reaction or response to each one. Some colours naturally make us feel more open and expanded, while others make us feel more contracted. We may also be reacting in a certain way because we are associating a colour with a previous personal experience. In the United States many hospital rooms used to be painted pale green. Since I spent long months in hospitals, I naturally had an aversion to that colour. Now, after a wide variety of studies on the healing effect of colour, those hospital rooms are being painted in different colour tones.

Our relationship to colour also can be an expression of what is happening in our energy fields as a result of an emotional reaction and mental decision to a situation or event. For example, if our first and second chakras are not balanced, the emotional reaction registered in our energy field is perhaps that we have lost our will to live and also our sexuality. By wearing red or orange to balance that chakra, it may bring forth emotional issues that are blocking the area, thus allowing the area to be cleared. Perhaps we have an underactive thyroid: blue supports the balancing and harmonizing of the throat centre as it expands. If the thyroid is overactive you can use green to balance the area, as perhaps there is too much blue in that centre. When working with colour there are no strict rules, but generally the chakras respond well to the following colours by chakra:

First Chakra (Root) – Red and Black

Red increases your connection to the earth and strengthens the basic will to live in the physical world. It is the colour of passion and will, good for all organs in root chakra area and the legs. Black helps you to come within yourself and be centered. It is a more masculine energy and can be like coming back into the womb or the void to find deep, internal creative forces. If used well, it can support and strengthen you. Overuse can bring depression. It is good for healing the bones.

Second Chakra (Sacral) – Orange

Orange stimulates the sexual energy and enhances the immune system. It increases your ambition and is good for all the organs in the sacral area. It also opens you to your creative expression.

Third Chakra (Solar Plexus) – Yellow

Yellow is good for mental clarity and a sense of what is just or fair. It is a warming soothing colour, like sunshine, and is good for all organs in the solar plexus area.

Fourth Chakra (Heart) – Green or Rose

Green promotes a strong active love for others, and healing for heart and lung problems. It helps you to love. Green embodies the balance and full-ness of love – everything is fine with me, you and the world; and nurtur-ing – think of Mother Nature. It is especially good for the heart and lungs and all the organs connected to the heart centre. Pink represents a soft, yielding love for others.

Fifth Chakra (Throat) – Blue

Blue helps you to speak the truth, increases your sensitivity, strengthens the inner teacher and brings peace, truth and a quiet sense of order. It is wonderful for all issues of trust. Dark blue helps put you in touch with a deeper sense of purpose and is good for all the organs in the throat chakra area.

Sixth Chakra (Third Eye) – Purple

Purple opens up spiritual perception, brings a feeling of ecstasy, and deep-ens your spiritual life. Purple promotes integration and movement into spiritual awareness, and carries a sense of royalty. It increases your sense of leadership and respect. Lavender promotes a lighthearted attitude to others and life. Purple encourages a feeling of 'lightness', and supports all the organs and glands in the third eye area.

Seventh Chakra (Crown) – White, Gold and Silver

White helps connect you to your purity and innocence. It brings spiritual expansion and connection to others on a spiritual plane. It reduces pain and is very good for the brain. Gold enhances the higher mind and your connection to God and the spiritual strength in you. It strengthens all parts of the body and has a masculine energy. Silver helps you to move faster and communicate better – 'quicksilver' (feminine energy).

Of course, there are many colours and tones of colour – always trust your intuition in choosing. You can place a coloured square of material or paper over the area of a chakra. Place your Reiki hand on top of the coloured square, sending the energy through the colour into the area. Using this method accelerates the balancing effect, which also seems to be deeper. If you have been attuned to Reiki Two energy, you can use that energy when working with colour.

You also can use the seven basic colours – red, orange, yellow, green, blue, purple and white – on the seven chakras and energize the crown chakra, using Position 2 for the head (see page 38). The energy goes through both sides of the brain, bringing about integration, and continues down the body to produce harmony in the entire body.

Use colour in your everyday life for harmony. Choose colours for your clothing and the rooms of your living space that promote inner peace and balance.

Reiki with Crystals

Crystals have different vibrational qualities, as well as colours. You can energize the balancing effect of crystals with Reiki. By placing your hand directly over the crystal as it is lying on the body, the healing effect is intensified. Each crystal has its own harmonizing effect and they are generally used in the area of the chakra. Remember that, ultimately, it is your intuitive nature that will guide you where to place the stones. Trust yourself and your Reiki hands. Of course, more than one stone can be used in any one area. I have found it beneficial to spend quiet time in meditation with each stone, to feel its vibration and to develop my own relationship with each one, before I use the crystals on other people. As to the cleansing of stones, there are many schools of thought. I use a simple prayer with each stone, saying, 'I dedicate you to the light of Christ. I programme you to be self-cleansing and to work for the highest good of all mankind.' Once you have completed a Reiki Two seminar, you can use the symbols from Reiki Two to clean the crystals. Crystals love the sunlight and like to be bathed and cleansed just like us. Some basic stones and their healing properties are listed below, by chakra.

Crown Chakra

Clear Quartz

When people think about crystals, pure quartz is usually the first one they think of. Quartz is known as 'the salt of the earth'. It is composed of silica – the most common mineral compound on our planet. The six sides of a quartz crystal represent the first six chakras. The sides come together in a point, symbolizing the seventh or crown chakra. This is our connection with the infinite. Most quartz crystals grow from a flat base. They are usually cloudy or milky in colour at the base and get brighter at the top – a symbol of our growth from shady beginnings to our brightest point, which connects us to the infinite in ourselves and to cosmic harmony. Quartz crystals, in their perfection, look like pyramids, which are also instruments that enable high frequency energies to come into physical reality.

Clear quartz reflects clear white light that can be directed to everyday thoughts, feelings, words and situations. Clear quartz has a tremendous ability to vibrate on the levels of colour frequencies (from black to yellow, from green to pink, and blue to purple). This demonstrates how clarity and cleanliness can enter into even the darker and lower frequencies.

These crystals prove that all the chakras can vibrate at once and still work together with light. Quartz can bring the aura to a very high frequency and, in this process, all colours of the aura get brighter.

Single quartz crystals are used for directing a stream of energy between the chakras. You just point the end of the crystal in the direction in which you wish the energy to flow.

Summary of Characteristics
Clear quartz: improves the crystalline characteristics of the blood, body and mind; activates and improves the functioning of the brain; excellent for meditation; works with all the chakras.

Milk quartz (white): helps with milk production; enhances bones and teeth; works with the entire body and all seven chakras.

Third Eye Chakra

Amethyst

Amethyst is a variety of quartz that strengthens the endocrine and immune systems. It enhances right brain activity and the functioning of the pineal and pituitary glands. It is one of the best stones for meditation, as it calms everyday thoughts, allowing the mind can be clear and focused. It is an excellent room cleanser and energizer. It transmutes our lower nature into higher potential. It cuts through illusion and enhances psychic abilities. It initiates the wisdom, humility and modesty that accompany a calm mind. It has an excellent calming effect. It is often used with rose quartz to clean the mind and console the heart.

Summary of Characteristics
Calming, strong protective qualities; for inspiration and intuition; strengthens the immune and endocrine systems; works on the third eye and crown chakras.

Throat Chakra

Blue Agate

Blue agate is a part of the quartz family that reflects the light-blue vibration that is most effective on the throat chakra.

We often have a program inside of us that puts a different perspective on our true spiritual selves. Many people's thoughts and feelings come from fear or lack of understanding and thus refusing others so that it causes imbalance in the throat chakra. When we do not express ourselves and feel restricted, the throat chakra becomes constricted and can cause headaches and imbalance in the throat. Because the throat chakra is located between the heart and head, the function of this chakra is to be a medium for the expression of our thoughts. By putting blue agate on the throat chakra it helps us to express truly our thoughts and feelings, both conscious and subconscious. This stone is also good for counteraction of red energies like passion, infections, inflammations and fevers.

Summary of Characteristics
Empowers the whole organism, especially the body and mind; gives the strength of goodness, courage, trust and clear communication; helps to clear away frustration and lassitude, as well as eye illnesses and breathing and nerve problems; works with the throat chakra.

Lapis lazuli

Lapis lazuli is a deep blue coloured stone, tinged with gold, that has always been a symbol of power and majesty. Traditionally, it symbolized God's energy and his mission on the earth. The Egyptians used a powdered form of the stone for cleansing the body of poisons and impurities. They also believed lapis removed demons. Today, this stone is used for mental and spiritual cleansing. It strengthens the skeletal system, and activates the thyroid gland, thus releasing tension and anxiety.

Summary of Characteristics
Encourages mental clarity and illumination, thus enhancing psychic ability; good for creative expression; a royal stone, to use with humanity and love; works with the throat and third eye chakras.

Sodalit

Sodalit strengthens the metabolism and lymphatic system, and balances the masculine/feminine polarities. It aids the pancreas and balances the endocrine system. It calms and clears the mind, thus alleviating fear. It cuts through density and illusion, bringing clarity and truth. It enhances communication and creative expression. It is slightly grounding and acts like a sedative. It works with the throat and third eye chakras.

Turquoise

The Native American Indians believe that turquoise is the messenger of peace, harmony and that it represents the energy of the grandfather. It attunes and empowers the whole body. It helps with the circulation of air and blood in the lungs, which in turn strengthens the whole respiratory system. It vitalizes the blood and stabilizes the nervous system. It is used for balancing the mind during meditation, and for promoting constructive expression, communication, friendship and loyalty. It is great for expressing the truth in every form and for encouraging a person to listen to their inner voice, that connection to the source.

Turquoise is sensitive to the touch and loses its shine if it is not used for a while. It helps a person to feel the calm of the blue sky and the emotional deep of the ocean and yet still be grounded. 'God's aspect prevails.'

Summary of Characteristics
Known as a 'happy' stone; tunes and empowers the whole body; helps with blood circulation in lungs; promotes peace to the mind, emotional balance, good communication and a friendly atmosphere; works with the throat chakra.

Heart chakra

Aventurine

Green aventurine is a member of the quartz family and reflects clear green light. It is used for many kinds of illness on the mental, emotional and physical levels. The clear green healing essence can help with all kinds of problems and has a calming vibration. It is good for the heart, as it counteracts emotions and gives greater balance to the physical body.

Aventurine can be used on any part of the body to reflect the healing green light into the aura. Aventurine crystals are recommended to wear when a person is stressed. Put aventurine near to the heart and solar plexus chakras to release deep emotional trauma and soothe stress.

Summary of Characteristics
Aids the release of anxiety and fear; strengthens the blood and stimulates muscle tissue; assists in purifying the mental, emotional and physical aspects; promotes emotional tranquillity and health; a heart healer; works on the heart chakra.

Chrysopras

When you hold Chrysopras it is like being in touch with the Mediterranean sea – slightly green with a white froth (foam) – gentle and calming. It is a member of the quartz family which moderates neurotic problems and depression. It harmonizes sexual imbalance. When used or directed to the heart chakra it dispels pain and sadness and brings inner peace. Chrysopras has a prevailing feminine aspect that fosters qualities such as gentleness, patience, tolerance, humanity and grace. It bolsters hormone regulation during the menstrual cycle and is good to use during pregnancy. It is also great for men to use, to help them with the ability to feel and heal emotional problems.

Summary of Characteristics
Regulates the hormone; provides support during pregnancy; moderates depression; gets people in touch with feelings; works with the heart and sacral chakras.

Malachite

Malachite aids the functions of the pancreas and spleen. It reduces stress and tension and aids sleep. It promotes tissue regeneration, and strengthens the heart, circulatory system, pineal and pituitary glands. It reveals subconscious blocks and vitalizes the body and mind. It works with the heart and solar plexus chakras.

Rhodochrosite

Rhodochrosite is often found with white lines running through a reddish, pink- to peach-coloured medium. It is used to clear the solar plexus and to integrate the energies of the physical and spiritual realms. It acts as a bridge for the heart, solar plexus and root centres, enabling the person to have a clear capacity for selfless love and compassion. As the bridging of these chakras takes place, the person is empowered in their physical aspect to utilize their full creative potential. It works very well with Malachite to clear and balance the chakras.

Summary of Characteristics
An emotional balancer, helping to heal emotional wounds and traumas; aids the spleen, kidneys, heart, prostrate gland and the circulation of the blood. The pink/red colour helps to blend the courage and passion of the root chakra with the loving expression of the heart. It is for divine love, and acceptance of yourself and your life. It works with the root, solar plexus and heart chakras.

Rose quartz

Rose quartz is a member of the quartz family that has a beautiful soft vibration and great healing potential. It promotes peace with its soft colour vibration. It is a stone for people who have not enjoyed life – perhaps as a result of not receiving or giving enough love. It helps to clear stored anger, resentment, fear and jealousy. People can be made to feel the real meaning of love with the aid of the pink light that this stone brings into the aura.

'After we can truly love ourselves we are able to love others without any prejudices.'

Summary of Characteristics
Helps kidneys and the circulation; increases fertility; calms sexual and emotional imbalance; helps to clear accumulated anger, and aids the development of forgiveness, compassion and love; works with the heart chakra.

Solar Plexus Chakra

Citrin

Citrin reflects a range of colours from light gold through to dark brown. Citrin's energy is similar to that of the sun – energizing, calming and life-giving. Citrin helps to increase creative power and define ambition. It is also excellent for use on the sacral chakra, which is the geometric centre of the body. If it is used for egoistic purposes, it can bring loss and sorrow to the person who misuses it.

For sensitive people, it is good to wear or carry citrin all the time. The yellow colour vibrations increase the amount of the light around the person and create an aura of security.

Citrin is great to use when we are trying to be successful in creativity, education and interrelationships. It brings the power of golden light into the material dimension of real life.

Summary of Characteristics
Excellent for the kidneys, liver, gall bladder, colon, all the digestive organs and the heart; can be used for tissue regeneration; a detoxifier for the physical, emotional and mental aspects; helps one to see clearly into one's personal problems; alleviates depression to bring about a sense of light-heartedness; works with the crown and solar plexus chakras.

Tiger's eye

Tiger's eye is part of the quartz family. It has a strong vibration that reflects a biscuit to dark-brown colour, which grounds energy into the roots of the Earth. This stone contains two different types of energy. The saturation of the brown background symbolizes the richness of the Earth. The delicate golden light is a statement of the crown chakra. With the combination of these energies tiger's eye is used to influence the solar plexus centre and to bring the higher sense of the crown chakra into physical reality. If you put tiger's eye on the solar plexus chakra, you can direct higher energy coming into the body to this area and create a sense of well-being.

Golden facial brightness reflects the eye of the tiger and symbolizes self-power, integrity and the ability to put heaven on earth. Tiger's eye can give an ability to see God in all his material forms.

Summary of Characteristics
Beneficial for the spleen, pancreas and digestive organs; has a grounding and centring effect that is slightly masculine in polarity; works with the sacral and solar plexus chakras.

Topaz

The colour of topaz varies from golden to blue to clear brown. It supports a clear stream of self-empowerment from the heart to the root chakra, enhancing our connection to the Earth. The greatest concentration of this energy is in the solar plexus: this is the area where our personal power is expressed. Our solar plexus energy is important to our life happiness. If this centre is constricted, then our ability to accept knowingly the way things are, or to be more flexible, is restricted. This stone ties God's or the Creative power into human acts, illuminating the higher self.

Summary of Characteristics
Vitalizes the liver, gall, spleen, digestive organs and the nervous system; extracts impurities from the body; works with the crown, solar plexus and root chakras.

Sacral Chakra

Carnelian

The red-orange colour of this stone is one of the most popular stones from the chalcedony family. These stones vibrate on lower frequencies than do quartz or amethyst. Carnelian is a symbol of the power and beauty of our Earth. Its colour is an expression of the golden-orange dawn, blush sunset, autumn leaves and richness of the Earth. Carnelian is used for grounding energy and is great for preoccupied people, or those who cannot concentrate and even get flustered. It focuses attention on the present moment, thus helping a person to concentrate better and be more productive. In meditation, it helps one to concentrate on higher goals. Its red-orange colour stimulates sexual energy and helps to clean blood in the reproductive organs. It empowers potency and pregnancy. Carnelian stimulates deeper love and the appreciation of the beauty and gifts of the Earth.

Summary of Characteristics
Stops bleeding and decreases fever; energizes the blood; helps with kidney activation, and with tissue regeneration in the lungs, liver, pancreas and gall; provides life to the physical and mental bodies, and connects the physical with the essential body; facilitates concentration, opens the heart and activates constructive energy; warm, sociable and joyful; works with the heart and root chakras.

Root Chakra

Blood Jaspis

Blood jaspis is a mixture of colours – green for the heart and red for the blood. Slightly masculine and with a cooling or warming effect (depending on what is needed), it is a strong instrument for cleansing the physical body. Jaspis cleans the blood and vitalizes the organs involved with the kidneys, liver and spleen. There is a big force that is hidden in this green/red crystal combination, with the healing green colour being directed into the bloodstream. For people that have been through mental or physical problems, jaspis can provide increased light and energy.

Summary of Characteristics
Strengthens the heart, spleen and marrow of the bone, by energizing and oxygenating the bloodstream; enhances physical and mental vitality and reduces emotional and psychological stress; aids in balancing deficiencies and links the heart with the root chakra; feminine energy that also assists in inner guidance; works with the heart and root chakras.

Obsidian

Black obsidian is connected to the root chakra. It acts like a magnet and brings spiritual power into the body and manifests the connection to outward expression. When you put it on the lower chakras, it magnetizes a soft, higher chakra energy, which makes the ego soft and clear. Obsidian teaches us the real meaning of the colour black – black is heavy, dark and unknown, the opposite to white, which is visible, light and known. The colour black is the master sign on the physical level. Wearing a black belt is a symbol of achievement of the highest level in the art of grounding and spontaneously using cosmic energy (chi) for self-defence. To be a success in life and emulate one of the living masters (Jesus, Buddha, Mohammed), a person must learn to overrule the self-centred temptation to impose power, and must not have a negative approach to the world.

111

Obsidian demonstrates the ability to remain connected with the light in the presence of the real world, and to keep a balanced mind in the rush of the twentieth century. Obsidian looks at all appearance from a neutral perspective, which helps us to discern the truth clearly. Black obsidian says that the sky is a mind condition that we can experience on earth by living in the real world. It attracts qualities of the soul into the body and purifies everything that has lower vibrations.

Obsidian is good for emotional people with a tendency to be distant, because it stabilizes unstable energies. Like other black stones, it needs to be used carefully – the person needs to be prepared for changes which they need to go through to get higher in their process. Obsidian is like a mirror that reflects mistakes and increases fears, insecurities and temptations to be self-centred that impede the higher soul qualities.

Summary of Characteristics
Supports the stomach and intestines; absorbs and eradicates negative energy; good for reduction of stress; masculine in nature; works with the root chakra.

Hematite

Hematite enhances personal magnetism, optimism, well-being and courage. You can put it on the third eye to reflect the subconscious, thus enabling an understanding of ourselves that is based on clear and creative positive thoughts. It is good to use after an operation, as well as for shocks, traumas and stressful situations.

Hematite can help people who have sleeping problems or who suffer from nightmares. Place the stone under your pillow to ground and stabilize the etheric body while sleeping. It has a direct effect on the bloodstream.

Summary of Characteristics
Excellent for the kidneys; activates the spleen; increases resistance to stress; helps with oxygen circulation; works with the root chakra.

Reiki with Meditation and Other Harmonizing Techniques

There are a variety of meditation practices which are all beneficial to the individual. If I am wanting clear vision into a problem with the stillness of my mind, I place my hands over the third eye area to energize and harmonize my intuition. If I am meditating on a question regarding trust and/or communication, I place my hand at the throat centre. Not only does the hand provide a focus, the energy actually helps the chakra to clear, thus enabling answers to come forward. I truly believe that the heart is our centre of knowing and that all our experiences are integrated through the heart centre. It is for this reason that I will often meditate with my hands on the heart centre. However you choose to integrate Reiki into your meditation, I am sure your experience will be enhanced.

Reiki can be used with any technique for harmonizing. It has been my personal experience to use Reiki with sound, colour, crystals, homeopathy, nutrition, flower remedies, accupressure, reflexology, psychological and spiritual counselling, regression therapy, massage, whole brain re-education, bioenergetics and psychotronics. You, as an individual, will take the best of what you experience and already know and combine it with Reiki to make it uniquely yours. Above all, we should realize that we are only the vehicle for divine unconditional love and that everything else is like the flavourings or seasonings that are added to it. It is my hope that, should you choose Reiki as a pathway for yourself, you also continue to find out more about yourself and our world using different techniques. Ultimately, all things are part of the greater whole, as we are one with all things in our world.

Chapter 10

The Endocrine System and the Chakras

In the teachings of Dr Usui and Takata, they stressed the importance of harmony in the endocrine system and of balancing the chakras.

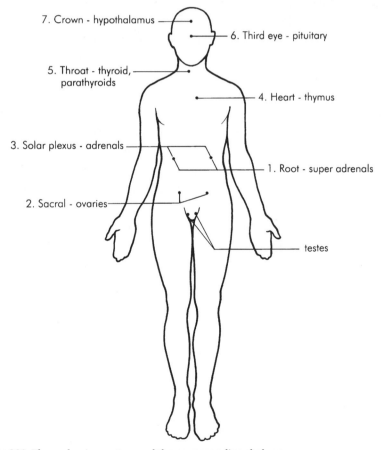

7. Crown - hypothalamus

6. Third eye - pituitary

5. Throat - thyroid, parathyroids

4. Heart - thymus

3. Solar plexus - adrenals

1. Root - super adrenals

2. Sacral - ovaries

testes

Figure 120: The endocrine system and the corresponding chakras.

The endocrine system and corresponding chakras:

7th Chakra	Crown	Hypothalamus
6th Chakra	Third eye	Pituitary
5th Chakra	Throat	Thyroid and four parathyroids
4th Chakra	Heart	Thymus
3rd Chakra	Solar plexus	Adrenals (cortex medulla)
2nd Chakra	Sacral/base	Testes in males, ovaries in females
1st Chakra	Root	Superadrenals

Although our endocrine glands have specific individual functions and work independently, overactivity or underactivity of one gland will affect the entire system. These ductless glands produce hormones, which are chemical messengers that pass into the bloodstream and circulation to stimulate or inhibit activity of other organs and tissue. Hormones regulate important processes of the body, such as metabolism, growth, aging, maintenance of stability of the internal environment (homeostasis), the body's ability to heal itself, resistance to stress and reproduction. Some other systems also produce hormones that are passed into the bloodstream: the digestive system produces gastrin in the stomach; enterogastrone, secretin, cholecystokinin and pancreozymin in the small intestine; and erthropoietin and rennin in the kidney.

The hand positions used in Reiki correspond to the location of the major endocrine glands in the body. The glands work together in harmony. Stress is the major inhibitor to the harmony of the body's metabolism. Full body treatments with Reiki reduce stress, allowing the body to heal itself naturally.

When using hand positions on the head, the energy is directly influencing the pineal and pituitary glands. The pineal gland is the major gland controlling the amount of light that is brought into the body, and regulates sexual development and skin pigmentation. The pituitary gland enhances the state of the mind; regulates sleep, growth and body fluids; works to sharpen the senses of smell and taste; and encourages the body to replace dead cells.

When you are using the hand positions over the throat area, the energy is directly influencing the thyroid gland which regulates the rate at which we burn up food and the rate of intensity at which we live. It keeps the iodine level correct in our body, regulates the mucous membranes, aids digestion and builds nerve and brain tissue. The energy also affects the parathyroid glands which regulate calcium levels in our bodies and promotes a sense of calm.

As we move our hands further down, the energy will directly influence the thymus gland which is also called the 'transpersonal heart'. The thymus gland produces 'T'-cells, one of the primary agents for the body to defend itself against disease. Dis-ease also corresponds to our state of mind.

When our hands are placed over the kidneys, the energy is also directly influencing the adrenal glands which stimulate our sexuality and creativity. They gives us energy and stamina and good muscle tone. When working over the reproductive areas the energy directly affects our sexual glands and regulates fertility and our emotional states.

The system works beautifully when it is harmonized. We feel alive and happy!

The Chakras and Their Related Function in the Body

Chakras are energy centres and serve as gateways for the flow of energy and life into the physical body. Each chakra is associated with the glands and organs in that part of the body. They react and respond to energy and vibration. The energy flow of the chakra can be in disharmony as result of imbalance or stress in the emotional, mental or spiritual aspect of an individual. This disharmony can eventually cause physical illness. The chakras can be balanced by placing your hand on the energy centre. This will bring about a release of the blocked energy, and a harmonizing effect takes place. When all the chakras are balanced, the chakras will feel the same.

I am giving you some information about the chakras. I have listed their location; function; the emotional energy associated with them; how we block the energy (our thoughts); the resulting body language indicating an imbalance in the area; organs and body functions controlloed by the energies; and what kind of disease or illness will occur if there is imbalance. In the succeeding chapter, I will discuss further the emotional causes of illness, by chakra.

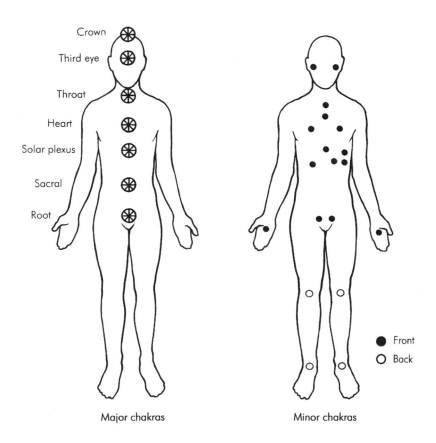

Major chakras   Minor chakras

Figure 121: The chakras.

The Energy Centres

1 Root Chakra (Muladhara)[1]

Location:	Where sacrum joins coccyx, in rear, to middle bottom of pubic bone, in front.
Function:	Seat of Kundalini energy; creative expression, abundance.
Emotional energy:	Survival; power; aggression; contact with the earth; the will to live; being active in the world; confidence; strength; self-acceptance; vitality; 'fight or flight' responses.
Blocks to these energies:	Fear of being in the world; feeling threatened in the above areas.
Body language:	Crossing our legs: our legs look all twisted up like a spiral.
These energies control:	Adrenal glands; kidneys; spine; joint controller of the bladder; affects the whole nervous system.
Diseases:	Problems of the legs, hips and buttocks.

2 Sacral Chakra (Svadhistana)

Location:	Between the pubic bone and navel.
Function:	Centre of sexual energy; feeling/emotional centre.
Emotional energy:	Sexuality; sensuality; personal creativity; nourishment; family ties; social behaviour patterns; sensitivity; social consciousness.
Blocks to these energies:	Feeling threatened in the above areas; lack of self-acceptance, self-love and self-esteem.
Body language:	Sitting with hip area back in chair and leaning forward; standing with hands clasped in front or behind.

These energies control: The gonads (ovaries and testes); fluid functions of the body.

Diseases: Reproductive disorders; pre-menstrual tension and irregular periods in women; impotence in both sexes; bowel and bladder problems; AIDS.

3 Solar Plexus or Power Centre (Mani Pura)

Location: Between the navel and base of the rib cage.

Function: Power and wisdom centre.

Emotional energy: Connections and attachments to people and things; love in attachment – dependency; relationship to the environment; draws in energy; expels stress; 'gut' feelings about people.

Blocks to these energies: Fears or anxieties about anything 'out there'.

Body language: Hands/arms over stomach area; legs crossed, elbows on knees; things on lap; hands hooked in belt.

These energies control: Adrenals; stomach; liver; gall bladder; the digestive system.

Diseases: Repressed energy at cell level, often leading to cancer; arthritis; problems with the above organs ('butterflies', constipation, diarrhoea, ulcers, digestive problems); migraines; heart disease in relation to our fear of power.

4 Heart Chakra (Anahata)

Location: Centre of the chest – sternum.

Function: Love, compassion.

Emotional energy: The whole: holistic thinking; impersonal feelings and unconditional love; healing centre; humility; responsibility; goodwill; tolerance; empathy and compassion. (The solar plexus is

119

selective and determines what you see – linked to one's belief system. The heart is inclusive and sees 'what is' – it picks up the soul quality of a person).

Blocks to these energies: The biggest aspect of the heart is unconditional love and trust of others. Therefore, blockages come from fear caused by old emotional hurts; lack of emotional security; fear of letting others in; and protection from recurrence of past hurts.

Body language: Arms folded; one arm across chest – holding books etc. there.

These energies control: Thymus gland; heart; blood pressure/circulation; the whole immune system; lungs.

Diseases: Heart attack; problems with blood pressure; problems of the circulatory system; immune system disease (AIDS).

5 Throat Chakra (Vishudda)

Location: Throat area.

Function: Communication.

Emotional energy: Creativity; self-expression; productivity; personal aliveness; individuality; action; desire for peace over conflict; trust of ourselves and others.

Blocks to these energies: Stifling of the above; rigidity; unwillingness to compromise; frustrated communication.

Body language: Coughs – clearing throat; wearing collar and tie, heavy necklaces etc.; hands on chin.

These energies control: Thyroid gland; voice; oesophagus; neck; lower jaw; strongly linked with Sacral Chakra.

Diseases: Diseases of the throat and lungs.

6 Third Eye or Brow Chakra (Ajna)

Location:	One inch above centre of eyebrows.
Function:	Intuitive centre; seat of will and clairvoyance.
Emotional energy:	Left hemisphere function (rational mind); integrated personality balance; planning – seeing into the future; will; purpose; control; self-control; ambition; choice; assertiveness; telepathy; super-ego – injunctions of parents; programmed actions, rather than appropriate responses. Right hemisphere function (creative mind); creative and artistic nature, the gentle, receptive, irrational and intuitive. It represents our relationship with feminine nature, both within ourselves and with others.
Blocks to these energies:	Confusion in any of the above areas.
Body language:	Wiping, rubbing and tapping of brow; hand on forehead when studying; furrowed brow when confused; eyes wide open when 'Aha' attained.
These energies control:	Pituitary gland – the master gland, controlling and balancing all the other glands in the endocrine system; nose; ears; sinuses; autonomic nervous system (linked with root chakra); hypothalamus; lower brain.
Diseases:	Diseases of the autonomic nervous system; hormonal imbalance; headaches; migraines; sinusitis; dizziness; depression; eye/ear problems.

7 Crown Chakra (Sahasrara)

Location:	Top (crown) of the head.
Function:	Connects us to our spiritual self.
Emotional energy:	Transpersonal awareness; the whole; systems; connectedness; relatedness; inner development; consciousness; unity with all things.

121

Blocks to these energies: Feeling cut off; alone (aloneness versus 'All-one-ness'); as all other centres come into balance, they are activated in the crown.

Body language: Hands over head; stroking hair back; hats; various religious practices of covering or shaving this chakra; crowns on kings and queens as a symbol of opening this centre and of unity with all things.

These energies control: Pineal gland (this gland is light sensitive, and is very active from birth until about seven years; secretes melatonin); time issues; circadian rhythms – jet lag effects.

Diseases: Serious psychotic disorders; being totally cut off, as in severe grief; deeply hurt people in psychiatric institutions; deep shock; inability to face reality.

[1] Names in brackets are the Hindi names for the chakras used in Yoga.

Chapter 11

Probable Emotional Causes of Illness, by Chakra

It is almost impossible to divide symptoms into individual chakras, as illness is interrelated. I have attempted to show you that, in each area, there is probable resulting illness. There are many more illnesses than those indicated, and many of these involve more than one chakra. Illness occurs when the energy is blocked in one or more of the centres. We should always look at ourselves and other people as whole beings: physical, emotional, mental, and spiritual, with the symptoms manifesting on different levels. It is safe to say that Reiki addresses the causes, as well as the resulting illness. This chapter is a way of looking at yourself and others to see what the probable emotional cause could have been, or is, in some cases.

Again, illness is the result of an imbalance, usually caused by a mental decision, based on an emotional reaction to an event or events in our lives. Once the mind is made up, then your life becomes an adventure of discovering how right your mind is, and experiencing the resulting illness which can, and usually does, occur.

Your mind is a powerful tool, which can work for and against you and your well-being. Reiki will enable you to clear the mind and open your heart to love and health.

This is in no way an attempt to list every illness or symptom of illness. It is merely a guide. Ask yourself: 'What are my thoughts and fears?', 'What am I not expressing, and how is this manifesting itself physically in me at this moment?' Your answers are always there inside you.

1 Root Chakra – Our Stability and Seat of Physical Vitality

Varicose veins: Usually indicates unhappiness in our choice of work; we feel overworked and overburdened.

Legs: Problems with the legs indicate fear of moving forward into life. If the upper leg is involved, it usually has something to do with past childhood trauma, which is keeping us stuck in a situation.

Kidney problems: Critical of yourself; a feeling of shame and disappointment in your life and in yourself. This is the place we store our pissed off energy and anger. Problems in this area usually indicate that this has not been expressed.

Knees: Knee problems are usually associated with our inability to be flexible, and involves our pride and ego.

Hips: Fear about going forward with major decisions; also the feeling of being unloved, and harbouring resentment.

Buttocks: This is a power or powerless indicator: soft buttocks can mean a loss of power.

Sciatic centre: Is usually concerned with being hypocritical; also a fear about money and the future. Holding on to fear keeps you from moving forward.

Anus: Can indicate guilt over the past and unwillingness to release the pain of it all.

2 Sacral Chakra – Our Centre for Sexual Energy

Lower back: Pain in this area usually means that you are not feeling supported financially.

Slipped disc: Feeling out on a limb, not supported by others in your life.

Appendicitis: Can mean that you are fearing life and blocking the flow of good energy.

Bladder problems: Holding on to old ideas, fearful of letting go; can also accompany anxiety.

Constipation: Stuck in the past; refusing to release old ideas and move on to something new.

Diarrhoea: Fear and rejection of things that may nourish you.

Female problems: A rejection of your femininity, associated with guilt and fear; can be a denial of your sexual energy.

Fibroid tumours/cysts: Usually occur after receiving a shock or extreme blow to your feminine ego.

Frigidity: Fear of pleasure: what will happen to you if you enjoy sex? Perhaps, also, insensitive partners.

Menstrual Cramps: You could be holding on to fear, thus creating tension in this area.

Miscarriage: Fear of the future – perhaps feeling it is not the right time; you are not ready on some level.

Pubic bone: Problems in this area usually involve genital protection.

Sterility: Fear and resistance to the process of life, and not trusting because of the fear.

Testicles: Represents the masculine energy and problems could result from a fear and rejection of this energy.

Vaginitis: Usually means that you are punishing yourself over sexual guilt, or that you are angry at your partner.

Venereal disease: Sexual guilt; in all cases of venereal disease, there will be an abstinence from sex and self-punishment.

Urinary infections: Usually being pissed off at the opposite sex or a lover, and blaming others.

3 Solar Plexus Chakra – Our Ego Centre

Adrenal glands: A feeling of being defeated, so that you no longer care for yourself.

Abdominal cramps: There is a fear, so you are stopping the process.

Appetite problems: Always fear; if you are eating excessively, you are feeling the necessity to protect yourself and are judging your emotions – eating instead of expressing; if you have a loss of appetite, you are usually not trusting life, and do not feel that you deserve to be nourished.

Belching: Fear that there will not be enough, so that you gulp life too quickly.

Diabetes: Holding on to deep sorrow, so that there is no sweetness left in life; also, a great need to control.

Fat/overweight: Probably running away from your feelings and protecting yourself; oversensitive to life.

Gallstones: So much bitterness and hard feelings that you have developed a condemning pride.

Gas Pains: These are usually undigested ideas, and you are gripped with fear.

Gastritis: Living with a sense of doom and prolonged uncertainty.

Indigestion: You have anxiety and dread; fear at the gut level.

Liver: This is the seat of anger and primitive emotions. Problems in this area usually indicate anger which has not been expressed.

Nausea: Fear and rejecting ideas and experiences.

Peptic ulcers: Fear and an overwhelming desire to please others, so that you become anxious.

Spleen: Being obsessed with things.

Stomach problems: Fear and dread that you do not have the ability to assimilate something new and unknown.

Arthritis: Overcritical and resentful; feeling unloved.

4 Heart Chakra – Our Centre for Unconditional Love

Asthma: Having the experience of being smothered by love; suppressed crying and the feeling of being stifled; you cannot breathe for yourself.

Anxiety: You are probably not trusting the flow of life and its processes.

Arteries: The arteries carry the joy of life: you are not allowing the full expression of joy in your life.

Back: Upper – stuck in all that 'stuff', needing to say 'get off my back'; feeling burdened.
Middle – feeling emotionally unsupported and unloved, and also not giving out love, holding on.

Blood: The blood represents the free flowing joy in your life.

Breasts: This is the mothering and nurturing aspect: you could be over-mothering, or have a fear of being nurtured or mothered yourself.

Lungs: Problems in this area usually mean that you have stopped receiving and lost the ability to take in life. Breathing problems represent the refusal to take in life in. Pneumonia means that you are tired of life, and desperate. These are emotions that you are not allowing yourself to heal.

Heartburn: There is so much fear in your life, that it is as if it is clutching your heart.

Heart imbalance: The heart is the centre for love and security; you are probably lacking joy, and have squeezed the joy out of your life; also indicates inability to love yourself and others.

5 Throat Chakra – Our Centre for Trust and Communication

Bad breath:	Contained thoughts of anger and revenge. Your experiences are blocked up and stale.
Blood pressure:	High – usually means long-standing emotional problems which have not been solved. Low – not feeling that you were loved as a child; a defeated attitude – giving up, as in 'What's the use?'
Bronchial problems:	Problems with receiving: breathing problems indicate a refusal to take in life fully.
Bronchitis:	Results from the family environment; an inflamed situation, and not expressing your sorrow.
Hay fever:	Emotionally congested with feelings of guilt.
Hypertension:	You have probably been fulfilling the needs of others, and forgetting about yourself; disappointed that you can not do what you want to.
Influenza:	This is your reaction to mass negativity and the fear around and inside of you.
Jaw problems:	There is so much resentment and anger, with a desire for revenge, that you become rigid.
Neck problems:	Your inflexibility and stubbornness have given you a pain in the neck.
Nose problems:	A crying out for love, and the need for self-recognition.
Teeth problems:	Feeling indecisive over a long time.
Throat:	Having the inability to speak up for yourself; swallowed anger, stifled creativity and the refusal to change.
Tonsillitis:	Fear and repressed emotion; not trusting of others or the future.
Thyroid problems:	A feeling of being humiliated: 'not what I wanted to do', 'when will it be my turn'.

6 Third Eye Chakra (Brow) – Centre for Extra-sensory Perception, Will, Purpose and Self-control

Arteriosclerosis: Refusal to see good – there is much resistance and tension.

Loss of balance: Not being centred, and having thoughts that are very scattered.

Lower brain: Incorrect beliefs, and the refusal to change old patterns.

Dizziness: Refusal to look; not wanting to be here; taking flight and running away.

Eyes: Represent your capacity to see clearly.
Far-sighted: fear of the present.
Near-sighted: fear of the future.
Astigmatism: fear of seeing your true self.
Cataracts: not being able to see the future.
Cross eyes: seeming to be at cross-purposes; not wanting to see what is out there.
Glaucoma: pressure from long-standing hurts; you are overwhelmed and unforgiving.
Wall-eyed: fear of looking at the present.

Ears: What are you wanting to hear? You are not being receptive to life around you.

Pituitary gland: This is your central control centre, your will; you may feel that you cannot control your thoughts.

7 Crown Chakra – Inner Development, Unity, Higher Consciousness

Brain function: The left side of the brain controls the function of the right side of the body. It has to do with logic, analytical and rational thought, intelligence, language and mathematics; corresponds to the masculine aspect, Yang. The right side of the brain controls the function of the left side of

129

the body. It has to do with understanding, creativity, feeling and intuition; corresponds to the feminine aspect, Yin.

Epilepsy: You are unable to accept your ability to be devoted, and feel that you are being forced in life.

Fainting: When you faint, you cut off the flow of life.

It has been my experience over the years, that if you have unresolved conflict, or issues with either of your parents, you can manifest physical problems in two areas:

Father: Left side of the brain; right side of the body; and the head.

Mother: Right side of the brain; left side of the body; and the legs.

There are several different therapies which address the imbalance of the chakras due to emotional/mental patterns: positive thinking, creative visualization and hypnotherapy. All are effective and can be used with Reiki.

Of course, there are many more symptoms that could be mentioned. There are any number of illnesses which involve several chakras. With Reiki, you do not have to know the cause, because the cause is addressed at the same time as the resulting physical problem. This chapter was written to give you more insight into yourself. It is my hope that you have benefited from it.

Wholeness is harmony: a perfect balance between our plus and minus aspects; masculine and feminine; giving and receiving; and being and doing. I believe that in this harmony and stillness, we can experience our souls and our oneness with all things.

Postscript:
My Personal Lesson for Living in the Moment, Trusting and Stepping Out in Faith

In October 1990, I was at an emotional and economic low. I was exhausted, physically and mentally. My visa to stay in the UK was about to expire, and I did not know where to go or what to do. My mind saw the doors closing on the UK as a sign that I was to go somewhere else. But where? If there was to be a change, what was it to be?

I prayed: 'Father, I know you are with me always. You guide my footsteps. Where am I to go and what am I to do to serve my brothers and sisters?' Ten minutes later, the telephone rang. It was my friend, Nick, who had just returned from Czechoslovakia. He said, 'Mari, you must go to these people: they need the message of peace and love that you bring.' I have long realized that God speaks to me through all beings. I had the answer to my prayers. My journey to Czechoslovakia was supported by another friend who gave me the money to go and said, 'I know that God wants you to go there.'

I began my journey to Czechoslovakia at the end of January 1991. I had just celebrated my 46th birthday. I was filled with excitement – the world seemed different. I was choosing to experience things in the moment, and to fully trust in God. When I arrived in Czechoslovakia, I had no money to live on. I could not have left even if I had wanted to. I remembered the message,

'Leave everything behind you and follow me. Trust in me.' Again I prayed: 'Father, please show me the way in which I can be of service to you. I willingly leave all things behind, to follow you.' An opportunity came to teach English in the local hospital in Kolin. The doctors there wanted to know what I really did, when I was not living in their country. It was the opening for their first experience of Reiki and of the unconditional love that this experience brings. The opportunity to teach Reiki in Czechoslovakia began. In the late spring, I taught the first class to the doctors and nurses of that hospital district in Kolin. I have been travelling and teaching Reiki all over the Czech Republic and Slovakia for the past six years. There are over eleven thousand Reiki students in that area alone. I have been to Poland, Norway, France, the UK, Austria, Germany and Greece and students have come from Russia, Switzerland, England and South Africa. There is now an International Association of Reiki, with three centres. The main organisation is in the Czech Republic, in Liberec. The other two offices are in Scotland and Poland.

The light continues to spread. Today and every day I give a prayer of thanks: 'Father, thank you for continuing to give me the opportunity to be of service to the world. I am a willing and grateful instrument for your divine love.'

My willingness to trust and to step out in faith has given me the ability to live my life more fully than I could ever have imagined possible. To be of service gives me the greatest joy. I am now 51. I am a mother and a grandmother. I have received a varied education. I have found that the best teacher is life itself. Life teaches me – I see and hear my Creator in all living things, and respond with love.

Come, join me…!

What is the Difference?

People have asked me why I chose this country to do my work and what the difference is between Eastern Europe and the West. First of all, I truly believe that the Czech Republic chose me. I responded to the messages I was given and, out of my vision, my work in Eastern Europe started here. It is very hard to put into words what I experience on a daily basis. There are so many sights, sounds and experiences that make up my relationship to this country and its people. The music stirs me to the very depth of my soul. Their songs are sung from deep inside – the oldest memories come to the surface. They sing about love, family, working in the fields and even drinking beer! – but with a joy for life that surpasses anything I have experienced before. I feel their hearts in their songs.

The country is beautiful – in spite of the environmental problems they are experiencing, there is a breathtaking beauty that is present. I love the villages with their own special character and the churches everywhere. It talks to me of a deep spiritual heritage and a pride in family and accomplishment. They are, as a group of people, independent, loyal, hardworking and fun-loving. They value their families and understand about commitment. They certainly have had opportunity not to believe they have an individual value, but that is changing and, as they value themselves more, others around them will value them likewise. They are innocent – there is a purity and cleanness present in them, as if they are unspoiled. I love seeing their eyes light up, with their spirit shining brightly. They are not afraid of hard work, and, when they decide to learn something, they put their entire being into the project. Small things are important to them. When they have made friends with someone, they are truly their friends for life. By their conditioning, they have for a long time been a society that does not trust. They did not trust the government, nor their neighbours. They only had their immediate family to be open with. They were taught that they did not really matter. What they thought or did was not important. I see that now they are finding that it does matter what they think and how they feel. They are part of the greater whole. The more they reach out and open up to people, the more there is potential for people to be open with them.

In the West, I find that people generally possess more material things, but that often it is the things that possess them. It has been a psychological game to see who can have more or better, as if that is how your personal value is established. It is by the external things the person owns that a judgement is made about their success or failure. I am not saying that this is true everywhere – but generally. The United States is so large, with many big cities. However, in the smaller communities it is probably not so prevalent. In their rush to develop technologically, people have moved away from the family. People often live so far away from each other that it may be years before the family is together. They move at such a fast pace that there is very little time to enjoy small precious

133

moments. They try to pack more and more into their day. I am speaking out of my own personal experience – I was like many Westerners. We perhaps do not know our neighbours well. On the one hand, we are more friendly at first – we greet people we do not know – so there is a informal attitude in many places. But we have a lot of acquaintances – and few close friends. In their search to find happiness, they take a lot of courses, but the majority of people are doing the course because it is the newest thing to do, so you hear 'Oh, I have done that' or 'I have been there'. Instead of integrating the material, it is more or less filed away. What is true? For the most part, people in the West know that their voices count, that what they think and how they feel is valued. They are hard-working people. The streets, contrary to belief, are not paved with gold. In most families, the mother and father both work to provide a living for the family. They have a big work ethic. The harder they work, the more they are rewarded. The more input they give to the job, the more they are valued as employees. So, if they are willing to work hard and believe in themselves and their contribution, they will reap greater benefits. People work hard and play hard as well. They are deeply committed to individual rights and the community. There are more and more groups of people coming together to address the environment, ecology and issues of society. They are interested in the world situation.

There are positive and negative aspects in both areas of the world. It seems to me that we can see and experience the polarity, one side having material things, the other not having. The not-having has enabled people to remain close to one other and make the most of everything. Please do not be so quick to reach for the other side. There is a middle road to travel for both the East and West, where I believe we can have our values of family, home, country and ourselves. Be willing to reach into the community and even out into our world. Be comfortable, but ever watchful of waste and the effects of our collective thinking and actions on our environment. Where we have our family structures, we are open, trusting and see what we share, rather than just our differences. It is all involves balance, just as Reiki is about balance. By being in the East, I have had the opportunity to experience the other side of the polarity at a very deep level, and to realize that here there is much more that speaks to my soul. The people here have been great life teachers for me. I am still learning from this country and the people. Here, I am more alive, more aware and happier with myself, and everyday I can see and appreciate the smallest things because I have the time to spend with those things.

Why Us...?

A long time ago, a group of people gathered with a spiritual teacher whom they called Grandmother. One evening, they asked her, 'Grandmother, what has brought us together this time?' She replied, 'We have come together to talk, from our hearts, about ourselves, our families and the problems of the world. We are all equal, and bring much to each other. At the end of the evening we must find our way home, so we reach to the central flame to take a spark of light, in order to light the way. But, remember that, not only do you light the way for yourselves, but you light the way for thousands of others as well. Hold your flame high!'

To all of you who have found this book and read it: there is a reason for our being brought together. We have been on a journey. May you always remember that you are the light of the world. Hold your personal flame high; show the others the way home to peace, understanding, health and love. I honour your search for the truth and a way to make a difference in our world.

Blessings and love.

Mari

List of Reiki Organizations

For many years, I found it unnecessary to belong to any organization connected with Reiki. However, my students in America, the UK and Holland wanted to join with their brothers and sisters in Czechoslovakia, so we formed the International Association of Reiki. It is a family organization, to support the awakened spirit in us all. The following are a list of the Reiki organizations of which I am at present aware:

International Association of Reiki – Main Office
Lesni 14
46001 Liberec
Czech Republic
Tel/fax: +42(048) 424629
E-mail: reiki@lbc.pvtnet.cz

International Association of Reiki – Scotland
The Reiki Healing Centre
Shawfield
Dunsyre
Lanark ML11 8NQ
Scotland

International Association of Reiki – Poland
ul. Igaňska 28
Warsaw
Poland

The Reiki Alliance
PO Box 41
Cataldo, ID 83810
USA

The Radiance Technique Association International Inc.
4 Embarcadero Center, Suite 5123
San Francisco
California 94111
USA

Reiki Touch Master Foundation
PO Box 571785
Houston
Texas 77057
USA

AERP Practitioners Association
27 Lavington Road
Ealing
London W13 9NN
England
(They also have a networking organization called: Reiki Visions, for which the contact person is Paul Dennis.)

There is also an organization called: Reiki Outreach International, of which the founder is:
Mary A. McFadden
PO Box 609
Fair Oaks
California 95628
USA
Tel: (916) 863–1500; Fax: (916) 863–6464
The organization was formed for the purpose of creating a network of Reiki channels who are united in service to humanity, and to the planet

137

Earth. Using Reiki daily, directing it to different situations and crises in the world, its aim and common purpose is to make a major contribution to world peace and harmony. The International Association of Reiki is the Czech representative.

European Contact:

Jürgen Dotter
PO Box 326
83090 Bad Endorf
Germany
Tel/fax: (08053) 9242

A Reiki Master does not have to belong to any of these organizations, but they generally do.

Bibliography

Arnold, L. and Nevis, S. *The Reiki Handbook*, PSI, 1982.

Baganski, Bodo and Shalila, Sharmon. *Reiki, Universal Life Energy*, Life Rhythm, 1988.

Baganski, Bodo and Shalila, Sharmon. *The Chakra Handbook*, Blue Dolphin, 1991.

Brown, Fran. *Living Reiki: Takata's Teachings*, Life Rhythm, 1992.

Hay, Louise. *You Can Heal Your Life*, Hay House, 1987.

Hay, Louise. *Heal Your Body*, Hay House, 1988.

Horan, Paula. *Empowerment through Reiki*, Lotus Light, 1992.

Jarrell, David G. *Reiki Plus First Degree*, Reiki Plus Institute, 1984.

Johari, Harish. *Chakras, Energy Centers of Transformation*, Destiny Books, 1987.

Lacy, Mary Louise. *Know Yourself Through Colour*, Aquarian Press, 1989.

Further Reading

Books

Arnold, Larry and Nevis, Sandy. *The Reiki Handbook*, Pennsylvania, PSI Press, 1982.

Baganski, Bodo and Sharamon, Shalila. *Reiki Universal Life Energy*, California, Life Rhythm, 1988.

Barnett, Libby and Chambers, Maggie. *Reiki Energy Medicine*, Vermont, Healing Arts Press, 1996.

Brown, Fran. *Living Reiki – Takata's Teachings*, California, LifeRhythm, 1992.

Burak, Marsha. *Reiki Healing Yourself and Others*, California, The Reiki Healing Institute Encinitas, 1995.

Elwood, Don. *Quest for the Light*, Virginia, FMB Publications, 1992.

Eos, Dr Nancy. *Reiki and Medicine*, Michigan, 1995.

Gleisner, Earline F. *Reiki in Everyday Living*, California, White Feather Press, 1991.

Haberly, Helen J. *Reiki, Hawayo Takata's Story*, Maryland, Archedigm Publications, 1990.

Hochhuth, Klaudia. *A Practical Guide to Reiki*, Australia, Gemcraft Books, 1993.

Horan, Paula. *Empowerment through Reiki*, Wisconsin, Lotus Light Shangrila, 1995.

Horan, Paula. *Abundance through Reiki*, Wisconsin, Lotus Light Shangrila, 1995.

Jerrell, David. *The Reiki Plus Practitioners Manual*, Tennessee, Reiki Plus Institute, 1992.

Lubeck, Walter. *The Complete Reiki Handbook*, Wisconsin, Lotus Light Shangrila, 1994.

Mackenzie Clay, A. J. *One Step Forward For Reiki*, Australia, The Reiki Teaching Centre, 1992.

Mackenzie Clay, A. J. *The Challenge to Teach Reiki*, Australia, The Reiki Teaching Centre, 1992.

Milner, Kathleen. *Reiki and Other Rays of Touch Healing*, Arizona, Milner Publications, 1994.

Mitchell, Karyn. *Reiki – a Torch in Daylight*, Illinois, Mind Rivers Publications, 1994.

Rand, William R. *Reiki, the Healing Touch*, Michigan, Center for Reiki Training, 1991.

Ray, Barbara. *The Reiki Factor*, Florida, Radiance Associates, 1983.

Ray, Barbara. *The Reiki Factor – The Expanded Reference Manual*, Florida, Radiance Associates, 1987.

Stern, Diana. *Essential Reiki*, California, The Crossing Press, 1995.

Stewart, Judy Carol. *The Reiki Touch*, Houston, The Reiki Touch Inc., 1988.

Veltheim, Dr John and Esther. *Reiki the Science, Metaphysics and Philosophy*, Pennsylvania, PaRama Publishers, 1995.

Articles in Newspapers and Magazines

Boginski, Boda and Sharamon, Shalila. 'Reiki – Universale Lebensenergie', Synthesis Verlag, Nov. 1985.

Graham, Vera. 'Universal Life Energy – Mrs Takata Opens Minds to Reiki', *The Times*, UK, 17 May 1975.

Hall, Mari. 'Universal Energy with Master of Reiki, Mari Hall from America', *Rude Pravo*, Czechoslovakia, 19 March 1992.

Hall, Mari. 'Reiki, not difficult but…', *Spirit* magazine, Czechoslovakia, June 1992.

Hall, Mari. 'Reiki, Universal Life Giving Energy, a Response', *Medium* magazine, Czechoslovakia, Nov. 1992.

Hall, Mari. 'The Message is Love, Reiki, the Instrument', *Regena* magazine, Czech Republic, 1993.

Hall, Mari. 'What is the Difference?', *Regena*, 1994.

Hall, Mari. 'Reiki with Other Therapies', a series of articles published over one year in *Regeneration* magazine, Czech Republic, 1995–1996.

Hall, Mari. 'Where There is Hope There is Reiki', *Vital* magazine, Czech Republic, 1996.

Hall, Mari. 'A Witness to Miracles', *Spirit*, April 1996.

Hall, Mari. 'Short Cuts – are They Effective?', *Regena*, May 1996.

Hall, Mari. 'Becoming a Master', *Vital*, May 1996.

Hall, Mari. 'Steps along the Way, a View of My Journey with Reiki', a series of articles for *Regeneration*, 1996.

In April 1996 Mari began writing a monthly column for *Vital* magazine, entitled 'In Your Experience', about integrating Reiki into one's everyday life.

Jacobs, Susan.'Reiki – Hands on Healing', *Yoga Journal*, USA, May/June 1984.

Zvelebil, Honza. 'Teacher of Reiki, Mari Hall', *Reflex*, Czechoslovakia, 18 Oct. 1991.

Zvelebil, Honza. 'Reiki – Mari M. Hall', *Regena*, Nov. 1991 – June 1992. This was a series of articles, including one on the hand positions used in the Reiki Manual.

Seminars

Mari writes and teaches a variety of seminars that are designed to support the 'awakened spirit'. She currently leads a nine-month seminar called 'An Adventure into Self-Discovery'; a five-day seminar, 'Life Cycles and Senses'; and intensive weekend courses on The Use of Crystals in Healing, Educating Your Whole Brain with Reiki, Meeting the Inner Child, Power Awareness, and Creating in the Now.

Journals and Newsletters

The AIRA *Radiance Technique Journal* is sent to all members of that
   organization.
The International Association of Reiki newsletter, *Heart of the Family*, is
   sent quarterly to all members of the association. It is full of information, support, news and experiences of the family.

Slide Lecture

Reiki, the Spiralling Energy, by Ingrid St Clare, London, England. I have not
   personally seen this slide lecture. However, Mrs St Clare is a well-
   respected Reiki Master, and is affiliated to the Radiance Technique.

This is in no way a complete representation of all the material that is
available about Reiki. It is merely an attempt to give you further avenues
for you to find out about Reiki, if it is your desire to do so.

Of further interest…

Creative Visualization

How to Tap your Hidden Potential

Ronald Shone

As children we all have natural imaginative powers, but as we grow up we are taught that these are 'unscientific' and 'illogical', and our ability to visualize creatively becomes obscured. Yet vivid imagery and symbolism affect us mentally, emotionally and physically, and while creative visualizations may not be logical – they may have the bizarre character of dreams or fantasies – they can radically transform our lives.

Tapping into this hidden potential can help us to define and achieve our goals. It can help us develop a positive attitude, raise our energy levels, overcome shyness and improve our memory. Exploiting the link between mind and body, creative visualization also enables us to fight pain and illness by participating actively in the healing process. Ronald Shone explains practical ways in which we all can make our mental imagery more potent and use creative visualization as a means of self-empowerment.

Author of the successful books *Autohypnosis, Advanced Autohypnosis* and *First Steps to Freedom*, Ronald Shone is Senior Lecturer in Economics at Stirling University.

How to Channel Healing Energy

Your Hands Can Heal

Ric Weinman

Because everything in the universe is made up of energy, healing energy can have a profound effect. The channelling of healing energy takes place when we allow ourselves to become a vehicle, or channel, through which the energy can flow. This energy can cure physical diseases by releasing the stress and long-held emotional traumas that are the root cause of disease.

How to Channel Healing Energy is a practical, accessible workbook of creative exercises that will guide the reader through three distinct methods of channelling. It shows us how to channel healing vibrations from sources in nature, such as colours, plants and crystals, explains how we can clear our chakras by aura balancing, and presents the subtle and esoteric art of Healing Through Oneness. Ric Weinman is an established teacher and healer who believes we all have the potential to learn how to channel healing energy to heal ourselves and others.

(Published June 1997)

The Chi Kung Way

Alive with Energy

James MacRitchie

'Chi' means 'energy' or 'life'. 'Kung' means 'working, developing or cultivating'. Chi Kung means working with your natural energy to be most fully alive. Until recently held in close secrecy in China and the East, this mysterious and wonderful ancient art is now rapidly becoming known in the West and recognized not only as an effective and enduring system for health and well-being, but also as one of the most exciting and important processes for achieving optimal performance and realising human potential.

The Chi Kung Way is a complete and comprehensive textbook, suitable both for the newcomer wanting to find out what Chi Kung is and how it works, and for the practitioner seeking more information. It translates Chi Kung into simple, straightforward language and includes practical instructions for 65 exercises which anybody in average health can do and enjoy, which will improve your quality of life and enhance your state of being in every way.

James MacRitchie has practised Classical Taoist Acupuncture since 1977 and has been teaching Chi Kung since 1983. One of the foremost Western experts and innovators in his field, he teaches and promotes Chi Kung internationally as an essential life-skill. He is the founder and Co-Director of 'The Body-Energy Center' in Boulder, Colorado.

Principles of Reiki

Kasja Krishni Borang

A comprehensive introduction to the Japanese healing system that is growing rapidly in popularity. This introduction explains:

- what Reiki is
- the different Reiki lineages and initiation processes
- what to expect from a Reiki treatment
- where to find a Reiki practitioner

Kasja Krishni Borang has been a Reiki master since 1984. She has taught Reiki internationally. Kasja lived in Swami Muktananda's ashram for six years and was initiated into the lineage by Vanja Twam. She is now based in the UK, where she runs regular workshops.

(Published June 1997)

Principles of Colour Healing

Ambika Wauters

Colour healing is a popular form of vibrational therapy. From ancient times healers and shamans, mystics and artists have used colour to heal body and mind. Colour affects our health, moods and behaviour and Ambika Wauters explains how to incorporate colour therapy into your life and explores:

- how colour healing works
- the chakras and their action
- how different colours affect you
- how you can use coloured light, water and food
- how to change your environment positively using colour

Ambika Wauters is a writer, healer and colour therapist. She is author of *Ambika's Guide to Healing and Wholeness – The Energetic Path to Colour and Chakras, The Angel Oracle* and *The Chakra Oracle*.
(Published June 1997)

Principles of your Psychic Potential

David Lawson

We all have the potential to develop our psychic and intuitive abilities. You may discover that you are a natural healer or a latent clairvoyant. You could awaken a powerful clairvoyant vision. Activating your psychic potential is safe, transformational and fun. This introduction includes:

- exercises to encourage your unique psychic abilities
- techniques for awakening your inner wisdom
- ways to develop the latent powers of your mind
- affirmations, visualizations and practical guidance to enhance your spiritual growth

(Published June 1997)

CREATIVE VISUALIZATION	1 85538 327 6	£6.99	☐
HOW TO CHANNEL HEALING ENERGY	0 7225 3471 X	£4.99	☐
THE CHI KUNG WAY	0 7225 3025 0	£6.99	☐
PRINCIPLES OF REIKI	0 7225 3406 X	£5.99	☐
PRINCIPLES OF COLOUR HEALING	0 7225 3340 3	£5.99	☐
PRINCIPLES OF YOUR PSYCHIC POTENTIAL	1 85538 487 6	£5.99	☐

All these books are available from your local bookseller or can be ordered direct from the publishers.

To order direct just tick the titles you want and fill in the form below:

Name _____

_____

Address _____

_____

_____

Postcode _____

Send to Thorsons Mail Order, Dept 3, HarperCollins*Publishers*, Westerhill Road, Bishopbriggs, Glasgow G64 2QT.

Please enclose a cheque or postal order or your authority to debit your

Visa/Access account – _____

_____

Credit card no _____

_____

Signature _____

– up to the value of the cover price plus:
UK & BFPO: Add £1.00 for the first book and 25p for each additional book ordered.
Overseas orders including Eire: Please add £2.95 service charge. Books will be sent by surface mail but quotes for airmail dispatches will be given on request.

24-HOUR TELEPHONE ORDERING SERVICE FOR ACCESS/VISA
CARDHOLDERS — TEL: 0141 772 2281